B10 00

D1079031

Evaluating Health Promotion

Edited by

David Scott
Institute of Education
University

Ros Weston
Research and Graduate School of Education
Health Education Unit
University of Southampton

Stanley Thornes (Publishers) Ltd

First published in 1998 by:
Stanley Thornes (Publishers) Ltd
Ellenborough House
Wellington Street
CHELTENHAM
GL50 1YW
United Kingdom

98 99 00 01 02 / 10 9 8 7 6 5 4 3 2 1

A catalogue record for this book is available from the British Library

ISBN 0-7487-3313-2

Typeset by Acorn Bookwork, Salisbury, Wiltshire
Printed and bound in Great Britain by T J International, Padstow, Cornwall

Contents

Part 3: Postscript

Contributors

Hein De Vries is Professor of Cancer Education in the Department of Health Education and Health Promotion at the University of Maastricht, The Netherlands. He is Director of Cancer Prevention Research Projects and his research and teaching interests include planning models, motivational determinants of health behaviour, health promotion interventions, diffusion and computerized tailoring.

Afaf Girgis is Deputy Director of Behavioural Science in Relation to Medicine at the University of Newcastle, New South Wales, Australia. She has published widely in international journals of psychology, health and medicine and is the current manager of a number of Australian evaluation projects.

Rob Sanson-Fisher has been Professor of Behavioural Science in Relation to Medicine at the University of Newcastle, New South Wales, Australia for the last 16 years. He is currently Director of National Cancer Control and continues to work in the field of health promotion. He has published over 200 articles, most of which have examined a variety of issues relating to improving health. He is a member of the International Union of Cancer Faculty on Behavioural Science.

David Scott is Lecturer at the Institute of Education, University of London. He has conducted a large number of evaluations in the fields of curriculum and health. He has published in journals such as *Forum, Curriculum, Journal of Policy Studies* and *Research Papers in Education* and in edited books. He has edited *Accountability and Control in Education Settings* and *Understanding Educational Research*. He is the current editor of *The Curriculum Journal*.

Keith Tones is Professor of Health Education at Leeds Metropolitan University. He is also a Senior Associate Lecturer in the Medical School of the University of Leeds and an honorary member of the Faculty of Public Health Medicine. He taught in a secondary modern school prior to working in teacher education for a number of years, primarily in curriculum development and the psychology of education. He launched the first post-graduate course for specialist health educators at Leeds Polytechnic in 1972, a course which is still in operation. He has published widely and is co-author of a popular textbook on effectiveness and efficiency in health education. His research has included investigation into the psycho-social and environmental determinants of breastfeeding, the role of health education specialists and the effectiveness of mass media on the prevention of skin cancers. He has acted as a consultant both in the UK and for the WHO and the EC. He has also worked with a number of universities in Europe. He is editor of the international journal *Health Education Research: Theory and Practice.*

Viv Speller is Senior Lecturer in Health Promotion at the University of Southampton. She joined the NHS in 1978 as a Health Education Officer and worked in a number of health education/promotion departments around the country, managing district-wide services in south London and Winchester. In 1992 she joined the Wessex Institute as the Regional Health Promotion Manager for Wessex and Health of the Nation Co-ordinator. Her particular interests in health promotion lie in developing systems to promote quality and effectiveness in health promotion and intersectoral working.

Ros Weston is Lecturer in Health Promotion at the University of Southampton. She formerly taught in comprehensive schools, further education colleges and many community education programmes through WEA. She was Lead Officer for Cancer Prevention at the Health Education Authority and then the UK Co-ordinator for the EC Europe Against Cancer Programme. She is a Fellow of the International Union of Cancer. She took up her post at Southampton in 1992 and since then has been responsible for research in evaluation for the Europe Against Cancer Programme. She has been a trainer and the Chairperson for Victim Support Wiltshire and is currently involved with women's health at the Salisbury Women's Health Centre.

John Wiggers is Lecturer in the Faculty of Medicine and Health Sciences at the University of Newcastle, New South Wales, Australia and co-ordinates the university's post-graduate courses in Health Promotion Studies. He has 15 years of experience in health promotion teaching, research and practice. Particular interests in health promotion research and practice focus on the provision of health promotion care by practitioners, socio-economic inequalities in health status and access to health care, and interventions aimed at reducing the extent of alcohol related harm in the community. His areas if teaching centre on the history and theory of evidence-based health promotion practice.

Acknowledgements

The editors wish to thank the European Commission and in particular the Europe Against Cancer Programme DG5, the International Union of Cancer and The European Cancer Leagues for the financial support for developing the research project which has resulted in the publication of this book. The research project was entitled 'The Mythmakers in Health Promotion: Is The Randomized Control Trial the Gold Standard?' and it resulted in a research report entitled 'Ways Forward for Evaluation of Cancer Prevention Programmes'. The editors have extended the research lessons learned to health promotion evaluation.

We would like to thank Karen Ragan who has typed parts of the script and organized the final product as well as communicating with all the authors and the publishers. Rosemary Morris gave both of us much support and encouragement at the beginning of this process and we are indebted to her. Last but not least, thank you to our families and partners who have constantly had to tolerate long working hours throughout the writing process and to all our colleagues in both the School of Education at Southampton University and the London Institute of Education.

Afaf Girgis wishes to communicate her thanks to Doctors Newell, Hancock and Perkins and to Professor Sanson-Fisher for their critical reviews of sections of Chapter 7; and to Ms Meiners and Ms Sullivan for their administrative assistance in preparing the chapter.

The authors and publishers are grateful to the following for permission to reproduce copyright material:
- Health education Authority (Figure 5.2)
- Health Education Research (Figure 4.3)
- Health Promotion Journal of Australia (Figure 8.1)

Every attempt has been made to seek permission to reproduce copyright material. We apologize if any have been overlooked.
- University of Southampton (Figure 2.4 and Tables 2.1, 2.2 and 2.3)

Introduction

Ros Weston and David Scott

This book has its origins in a recently completed research project, *'Ways Forward for the Evaluation of Cancer Prevention'* funded by Europe Against Cancer, directed by Ros Weston. In this project she used triangulated approaches to help her understand and cognitively map the world of evaluation. The three elements of this study were:

1. a discourse analysis of health texts to understand better the historical and paradigmatic shifts in health promotion/evaluation as well as the dominant models and approaches;
2. a systematic review of the literature of evaluation and cancer prevention/health promotion evaluation;
3. interviews with key leaders in the international arena of health evaluation.

She brought together the European Cancer Leagues at Chilworth Manor, Southampton, UK in December 1996 to enable them to study the findings and to explore how they might apply these to the evaluation of their health interventions. This resulted in an EU research report (Weston *et al.*, 1997) entitled *'Ways Forward for the Evaluation of Cancer Prevention'*. Though the various contributors to this book were prominent in this study, this does not mean that they share a common perspective. Indeed, what characterizes the field of health promotion evaluation is a diversity of views and a variety of epistemological frameworks, which are reflected in the contributions to this book.

The purpose of this book is to stimulate debate about how evaluators might work together to improve their knowledge of health promotion and better fulfil the aims of the World Health Organization's initiative Health for All (1986). At the same time, the book seeks to challenge the dominance of any one approach to evaluation and suggest that evaluators need to value and work with difference; that is, value the use of multi-methodological approaches in helping assess the effectiveness of health promotion. This challenges the exclusive reliance on either empirical or phenomeno-logical approaches, arguing that neither of these alone can provide a complete answer. We also suggest that such polarization is not really about evaluation but about the need for professional, personal or paradig-matic power and dominance. On the other hand we challenge this too and suggest that only through such confrontation, explanation and exploration are we likely to bring about positive change in the way we evaluate health promotion. This book therefore offers a number of different viewpoints. It is, however, intended to be used as a whole rather than as eight separate texts (edited papers which stand alone), moving as it does from an histori-cal exegesis, through an examination of methodological and ethical issues, to a discussion of the various perspectives and debates concerning health education. Each chapter does, of course, stand alone too.

The authors have all worked in this field for a number of years and each has created a 'text' and a discourse which is therefore grounded in their personal/professional research paradigm, personal values, ethics and their understanding of the social world. Their choice of evaluation metho-dology and method, purpose and activities is related to their interpreta-tions of this social world and the 'meaning/s' it has for each of them. Of paramount importance, and independently of these individual texts and discourses, there is agreement that evaluation of health promotion activity is essential. There is agreement too that it should be a part of the planning process, multi-methodological and illuminating as well as offering the 'best available information' for health strategists, policymakers, planners and practitioners. In addition, there is agreement about the need for research to elicit 'meaningful' information which remains grounded in reality and which is judicial – that upon which most reasonable people would take action.

A second area of consensus is on the role of evaluation in complex settings such as communities and the shortcomings of positivist/empirical approaches for usefully understanding this. In other words, there is a need for more sophisticated means of illuminating what actually happens in a programme/intervention and the meanings it has for those involved.

A third area of consensus is that evaluation is a 'structured and planned' activity which is part of the whole process and not just an 'add on' at the end which has often been seen to justify why a project took place and been overgenerous and less than critical about its success or otherwise. These approaches also challenge idiosyncratic and whimsical planning and development which tended to be the norm in the early years of health promotion.

A fourth area of consensus is that there is a need for cost-benefit analy-sis to be included in such planning as this may indeed show that health promotion is effective in ways other than just reducing risk, morbidity or mortality; that health promotion/education is indeed adding years to life and to the quality of life in ways we may still be novices in exploring and interpreting.

A fifth area is that evaluation needs to pay attention to both theory and practice. Understanding how the hermeneutic process operates to enable what is learned in practice to be tested theoretically and then tried in practice and how theory-in-practice can contribute to theory-of-practice are essential elements of health-promoting activities. It is therefore a multi-methodological activity with evaluators assuming specific roles in specific settings at given moments in time. As such, it cannot, however, be extricated from its own inter-relationship with other historical, economic, social, educational and cultural texts. Understanding this intertextuality may help evaluators to clarify and illuminate what it is they do and the worlds in which they do it and to understand more effectively the relations between the two. Reflexivity is therefore essential in understanding the role and purpose of evaluation.

The book therefore aims to:

- explain the various frameworks which have been developed for evaluating health promotion initiatives and interventions;
- make a judgement about their efficacy, validity, reliability and usefulness;
- locate the various models within social, political and epistemological frameworks;
- discuss successful and unsuccessful evaluations of health promotion initiatives and interventions;
- enrich debates about quality assurance, ethics, policy and knowledge concerning these interventions and initiatives.

The book is divided into three sections. Part 1 examines issues of history, process and quality. Part 2 discusses planning and evidence-led approaches. Part 3 focuses on two important areas: the ethics of evaluating health promotions and the theory–practice relationship.

In Chapter 2, entitled 'The historical context of evaluation in health promotion', Ros Weston charts the historical paradigm shifts in evaluation and therefore the knowledge/power dyads inherent in them. These have bedevilled both the evolution and evaluation of health promotion. She does this by deconstructing the various texts and discourses and shows by her research how such an analysis can illuminate theoretical and ideological debates. These may often dominate, in terms of fashionable methodologies and methods, the way both theoreticians and practitioners choose to work. She discusses the importance of having some consensus about evaluation and a planning process for ensuring it is an ongoing element of all health promotion work.

In Chapter 3, David Scott suggests that research methodology and in particular positivist/empirical approaches are inappropriate for much health evaluation. By problematizing these aspects, he argues against current dominant ideologies, particularly evidence-based health promotion. His argument is premised on the complex nature of the social world and social interaction, in particular that social actors are engaged in processes of interpretation all the time. In addition, he suggests that evaluative practice cannot be solely ethnographic. All methodologies have their problems and these are related to the relations between evaluators, stakeholders and the organizations being evaluated.

In Chapter 4, Keith Tones expands upon these issues. He disentangles the complexities of relations between knowledge, attitude and behaviour as well as the proximal/distal learning chain involved in the 'process' of health promotion. He deconstructs the 'objectives-led' approach and then illustrates how important objectives are in monitoring progress, linked as they are with outcome objectives. These are related directly to 'outcome' measures and the development of 'indicators' enabling the intervention process to be monitored over time and allowing comparisons to be made. He takes issue with cost-effectiveness/cost-benefit models and suggests that they rarely account for all the ways by which judgements are made about the success or failure of interventions. He makes a plea for the use of triangulation and suggests such an approach will help in the collection of 'judicial evidence' which will usefully inform future theory and practice.

In Chapter 5, Viv Speller concentrates on developing quality assurance programmes. She illustrates the importance of these for health promotion work as well as explaining how evaluation might be seen as a continuum rather than a set of polarized activities each with a different and often competing purpose. She makes a plea for more appropriately planned evaluation, including quality assurance and ongoing monitoring of the progress or otherwise of interventions and other activities. Quality assurance, she suggests, should take place alongside both process and effectiveness research and can be linked to the use of criterion-referenced or indicator systems which use outcome as well as process data.

Part 2 opens with a chapter by Hein De Vries in which he focuses on the planning cycle and shows how important it is to develop interventions which are driven by appropriate evaluation strategies. He argues that evaluation is an integral part of this planning and therefore challenges the view that evaluation is some form of 'add on' activity at the end of an intervention. He suggests that the use of such planning models allows researchers and practitioners to focus on important issues at the developmental stage of an intervention, thus reducing the possibility of failure and increasing the potential for efficacy.

Afaf Girgis, in Chapter 7, uses her experience in behavioural science to explore issues relating to methodology, especially with regards to evaluations conducted in complex settings. She illustrates by the use of case studies (grounded in actual intervention research) the importance of conducting needs assessments and of developing appropriate research designs. She demonstrates the learning inherent in such approaches and explains how it may enhance the planning and evaluation of health promotion.

Chapter 8, by John Wiggers and Rob-Sanson Fisher, examines the need for systematic approaches to the evaluation of health promotion. They suggest that, as in other areas of health, there is a need for evidence-based practice in the field of health promotion. Without such evidence, scarce resources are likely to be inappropriately allocated, resulting in inequities not only for those who receive health promotion interventions but also for those deprived of these efforts. Unfortunately, much of the practice of health promotion has not been rigorously evaluated due to a combination of factors, including a lack of skill and training of those in the health promotional field, a lack of resources being allocated to this area and a lack of sustainable funding. However, the need for such activities is being increasingly recognized and strategies which can be used to undertake such evaluations are being developed. While randomized control trials remain the gold standard, it has to be acknowledged that new designs need to be developed and evaluated if health promotion is to progress in a satisfactory manner.

David Scott demonstrates in Chapter 9, by drawing on the work of Seedhouse (1988), that the adoption of an ethical stance is crucial to the research process and, indeed, the researcher/practitioner relationship. It is equally important for evaluators. He challenges evaluators who promote evaluation as an 'objective science' which is rational and logical, arguing that they help construct the social world and need to recognize that they do so. Conscious reporting of bias is insufficient, which means that reflexivity is necessary for evaluators to be aware of the choices they make. It is also necessary in the sense of understanding the intertextual nature of all the work done in health promotion. These choices are not easy but relate to underlying 'meanings' about people, communities and societies. They illuminate the ongoing dynamic between social structure and social agency which makes the task of evaluation uncertain.

Finally, in the Afterword, we discuss the important relationships between theory and practice and theoreticians and practitioners. We suggest that only by learning to value all the different approaches, and to acknowledge that there cannot be one authoritative model, can we hope to understand what we do and how we do it. Understanding our successes and failures and learning from them may enable us to further our goal of positive health for all.

NOTES

Superscript numbers within the text refer to notes at the end of the chapter.

REFERENCES

Seedhouse, D. (1988) *Ethics: The Heart of Health Care*, Chichester: Wiley.

Weston, R., Farley, P., Fleitmann, S. *et al.* (1997) *Ways Forward for Evaluation of Cancer Prevention*, University of Southampton, Southampton.

World Health Organization (1986) *Ottawa Charter for Health Promotion*, Copenhagen: WHO Regional Office for Europe.

Intertextuality: the current historical context of health promotion, cancer prevention and evaluation

2

Ros Weston

For many years there has been an ongoing debate about the most appropriate ways to evaluate health promotion. This could be said to have reached its peak in recent times because of political and economic pressures as well as a paradigmatic shift towards evidence-based approaches, grounded as they are in both the empiricist (logical/positivist) research framework and the medical model of health promotion (Cochrane, 1972; Nutbeam, 1990; Weston, 1977). The concentration on an evidence-led health service has focused attention on both the nature and purpose of health promotion and whether or not it is effective. This changing economic and political panorama (the world view) can give the illusion that this debate has reduced health promotion, and indeed medicine, to nothing more than the saving of resources and the costs of health care, the human issues being subjugated in favour of a market-led economy in health – the 'supermarket of health' (Blair, 1997).

In terms of preventing disease, it suggests that the endpoint of all health promotion, the only appropriate measure of effectiveness, is reduced mortality, morbidity and risk. This is contrary to the WHO Alma Ata declaration that Health for All is about positive 'health gain' and not only the reduction of illness and premature death (WHO, 1946, 1978, 1984, 1985, 1986, 1992; Minkler, 1994; Tones and Tilford, 1994). In other words, rather than focus on the long-term nature and tasks of health promotion, that of enhancing positive health and health opportunities as outlined in the WHO Health For All programme, effectiveness is demonstrated only by whether mortality, morbidity and risk from specific chronic diseases have been reduced. Or, in community interventions, whether such measures as the introduction of seat-belt legislation has reduced the number of road deaths and injuries. Some research would suggest that this reduction has been achieved at the expense of more serious injuries because people drive faster, the seat-belt giving them the illusion of safety, yet this is still seen as the appropriate policy (Sanson-Fisher, 1985, 1991, 1993a,b; Sanson-Fisher and Redman, 1986; Sanson-Fisher and Byles, 1990; Sanson-Fisher and Turnbull, 1993; Sanson-Fisher and Campbell, 1994; Sanson-Fisher et al., 1992, 1993; Weston, 1997). The principles of the WHO programme go far beyond such an approach in that they seek to enhance health policy in order to create equity and opportunity for all people; to offer all people the opportunity of making the healthy choice the easy choice (Nutbeam, 1990; Minkler, 1994; Tones and Tilford, 1994; Weston, 1997).

How, then, can this change of emphasis be understood by both those working in health promotion and those in the business of creating theory and testing both theory and practice, the theoreticians in the research and policy institutes. It is so easy, and forgivable, for those new to health promotion to be moulded by the latest fashion and rhetoric as they may not have the historical perspective which enables them, whether practitioners or theoreticians, to see the major fashionable shifts (paradigm shifts) which have taken place over the last 25 years. Health, like education, can be a political and economic football, played, dribbled and manipulated constantly with the specific aim of scoring the winning goal, by politicians and those seeking power within the profession itself (power and knowledge dyads which are inherent in these paradigm shifts, Fox, 1993). Indeed, it is pertinent to question whether or not all that is achieved is an own goal. Through the Cochrane Collaboration there is the search for evidence, the possible 'truth': the best way to treat, operate, care or to health-promote.

Paradoxically what seems to be happening is that there is very little evidence to support much of what takes place in medicine, healing or health promotion. There appears to be no 'truth'. There is also the own goal of health promotion bringing about its own demise because the search for 'proof' that it works is turning out to be equally elusive. It seems that there is currently no research instrument specific enough to convince the economists, positivists and politicians that maybe it does work. If health promotion was to be defined more appropriately by using different endpoints, such as health gains, it may be found to be working very well indeed (see Chapter 4). It is not so easy to see how those who have been in the profession for some time could be quite so easily moulded and led. Arguably, they could be said to have very short memories. Or for reasons which can be extremely complex, being a mixture of the pressure from organizational change (driven by politics, economics and ideology), economic necessity, personal choice or otherwise, they have had to make theoretical or practical choices (shifts) against their better judgement. Or, they have made these shifts because they believe that recent research and practice knowledge, intertextually woven with economic, political and historical/social/cultural contextuality, have indeed proven that such a change is necessary and right. It is both a timely and appropriate change and one that will benefit health promotion in the long term. In other words, it will achieve the objectives of the Health For All programme.

How can this dialectical position be examined? This author suggests that it may be helpful to study/restudy the texts of health promotion and the associated discourses developed within these texts. This can illuminate the consequent interplay of those texts one on another (intertextuality) which will enable both practitioners and researchers to see historical paradigm challenges/shifts and the rhetorical (persuasion) and sometimes the ideological (perhaps misleading although not necessarily deliberate) devices which have given these their power/dominance at historical points in time. It can also illuminate the intertextuality of the research/evaluation and evaluation/health promotion debate and is thus enabling in that it can demonstrate that they are inextricably linked (Weston, 1997). To do this, it is necessary to fictionalize the texts as by so doing it is possible to 'linger in the texts' (Eco's 'lingering in the woods') and use a framework for analysing the discourses (the way the 'story' is told), clarify who is telling the 'story', classify the main characters in the 'stories' as well as being able to place these characters in a research or practice paradigm (the one/s that most often appear to underpin their work).

This allows the researcher and reader (Eco's (1995) notion of model authors and readers) to suspend belief, first in the present approaches to health promotion and subsequently in any models and approaches, in order to review them anew and allow them to tell their 'story'. Such exploration and illumination is dialectical in the sense that by allowing the various stories to emerge anew, reflexively, aspects may be revealed which hitherto were clouded by the researcher's/practitioner's own prejudice, rhetoric/ideology, training or lack of understanding. Or it could be that researcher/practitioner judgement was clouded by unconscious bias about the (autobiographical) creation of the theory/practice world (world-making). Or in another sense, and more importantly perhaps (moving from the autobiographical), such a world view may illustrate the lack of awareness of how the texts and thus intertextuality inadvertently promoted dominant paradigms and thus knowledge/power dyads which have remained, in large part, unquestioned over the last 20 years or so. As Popper (1959, 1969) suggested, it is only when worlds merge (or collide) that real debate begins to take place. He suggests that scepticism can be healthy in that there is a need for constant questioning in all 'worlds', something being 'true' only until it is proved 'untrue'. Phenomenologically speaking, this is the nature of all debate, ongoing over historical time, a constant dialectical dynamic. This chapter seeks to illustrate the intertextuality of evaluation, research, health, politics and economics and attempts to show that textual and discourse analysis can be an illuminating research tool for understanding the role of methodology/method in the evaluation of health promotion and also for questioning the nature and tasks of health promotion and the intertextuality of the one with the other.

WHAT CAN BE LEARNED ABOUT EVALUATION IN HEALTH PROMOTION FROM TEXTUAL AND DISCOURSE ANALYSIS?

The research upon which this chapter is based was carried out for the Europe Against Cancer Programme (Weston, 1997). It has charted the development of these debates and illustrates that professionals often have preconceived ideas about evaluation which remain grounded in their original professional and disciplinary training and their preferred stance about the behaviour of communities and individuals. This relates directly to their training in research and whether it was empiricist or qualitative in nature. Other key researchers (Nutbeam, 1990; Green and Kreuter, 1991; Steckler *et al.*, 1992; Evans *et al.*, 1994; Baum, 1995; MEANS, EU 1995; Weston, 1997) have illustrated that appropriate evaluation, particularly in complex settings such as the community, requires multi-methodological approaches and should be based on the principle of using the most appropriate research methodology/methods to answer the evaluation questions rather than the research methods researchers most prefer and are comfortable with.

In this world of health promotion as Weston (1997) argues, the choice of evaluation method is also related to the preferred model or approach practitioners and researchers use in planning and delivering health promotion. As can be seen in Figure 2.1, models of health promotion and evaluation methodology/method can be located in particular models of health and vice versa. There is some evidence that another model or approach is developing in its own right, that of effectiveness (see Figure 2.2).

So, there is an open debate about the nature of what constitutes appropriate evaluation in health promotion. However, there is some evidence that the debate risks closure through the pressure of the economic and political discourse of effectiveness and its associated claims to knowledge and power (Weston, 1997). It is important to expand on this theme a little. Recent appointees to health promotion may be forgiven for not

The Biomedical Model
This model is grounded in the principles of medical science such as:
- public health medicine;
- epidemiology;
- the body as an object entity.

The criticisms of this model are that it:
- separates body and mind, it is mechanistic;
- is iatrogenic, it can cause illness;
- is controlling, controlled by professionals who know best, therefore authoritarian;
- treats human beings as passive.

The Prevention Model
This model is grounded in the principles of medical science but with a recognition that education and information programmes are necessary to increase compliance, that is, to encourage more people to take advantage of health interventions. There is a move to a more interactive relationship with patients, individuals and communities.

The criticisms of this model would be that:
- it is paternalistic; caring for people who might not otherwise care for themselves, rather than promoting independent action;
- individuals can be seen as passive by professionals who know what is best for them.

The Education Model
This model is grounded in the principles of *educere* – to lead. Such practice would encourage:
- the interactive sharing of knowledge and information with individuals or communities;
- the educational process beginning where the individual or community is currently and not from the professional point of view or belief;
- choice making, which is voluntary, therefore individuals may not necessarily make the choices the professionals want;
- individual communities to develop their skills for changing behaviour, lifestyles, aspects of their current life condition;
- the exploration of attitudes to health, illness and lifestyle to enable people to review why and how they act about their health;
- giving of the relevant knowledge at a time when people are ready to receive it; in other words, at the point of motivation when they are most likely to act on such knowledge;
- continual maintenance for such action, especially at possible stressful times such as relapse;
- self-esteem, autonomy and individual control: empowerment;
- the professional being seen as a facilitator who works in partnership with people.

The criticisms of this model would be that:
- such practice is hard to measure because the reality in which it takes place is complex;
- it can be viewed as esoteric;
- much success rests on the uptake of knowledge and therefore action of the recipients;
- voluntary choice has drawbacks as individuals may not make the healthy choice, and therefore not comply with the views of health experts;
- it may not lead to concrete reduction in mortality and morbidity measured from the medical perspective;
- many assumptions about success can be made in the absence of planned evaluation.

The Community Development Model
This model is grounded in an integration of the Prevention and Education models. It recognizes that human beings can be active on their own behalf but that legislation may be necessary to improve health on a more macro level, for example seatbelt laws and immunization programmes. These both acknowledge the voluntary concept but to protect all people (beneficence) sometimes legislation or agreed codes of conduct are necessary.
This model:
- seeks to empower communities and recognizes differences in culture, economic and political realities;
- empowerment may be necessary to change the normative states; this may be achieved through self-empowerment or community empowerment, a good example being 'no smoking policies' in public places.

The criticisms of this model would be:
- that legislation is necessary to protect the majority of people – the concept of beneficence;
- that many would doubt the need for this;
- that the hidden agenda is to bring about a new normative state, where people will see healthy lifestyle and communities as the norm and those who do not conform will be seen as deviant.

The Radical or Political Model
This model seeks to change the nature of societies by health policy development. It seeks to provide:
- equity;
- justice;
- human rights for all people in all nations;
- positive health in an environment which has the conditions for such positive health: 'healthy public policy'.

It challenges governments to provide health-promoting environments and it therefore encourages the use of the most appropriate frameworks/models to achieve this. In practice this means a combination of all the frameworks described in this figure. Decisions about which one to use are based on needs assessment research, epidemiological data and professional knowledge and expertise.

The criticisms of this model would be that:
- equity is impossible for all nations as the wealth of some nations depends on the poverty of others: the global economic arguments;

- it promotes victim blaming when conditions of economic restraint, political ideology and the lack of a health-promoting environment exist, sometimes referred to as health fascism;
- it does not challenge the lack of human rights in some nations, but rather accepts them. This is a double-edged sword because if we accept that health promotion begins where the individual or community is, then this also applies to nations where we feel the conditions are not acceptable.

This model seeks to:
- bring about pressure for change in all societies from within the society itself;
- raise awareness of the need for a public health policy to enable positive health.

It could be argued that this is the world view of the author and that there are many other world views. In her opinion all other models can be superimposed on these, or vice versa, and the same spheres of action will be apparent.

Figure 2.1 Health promotion models.

realizing that many forms of evaluation exist other than the evidence-based effectiveness model grounded in the empiricist paradigm (logical positivism). Those educated in the last 20 years may not be aware of such political agendas (as these may be the only ones they know). Such agendas can be detected in the 'texts' of health promotion. One aspect of this research reveals that the 'story/ies' are those which the authors/ researchers wished to tell and these relate to their original disciplinary training and values and yet paradoxically these are also developing narratives (Giddens, 1991) which emulate work from a number of other disciplines and fields. Historically, the debate about methodology ebbs and flows with changing political, economic, cultural, social and educational texts and therefore the fashion in theory and practice does so as well. Within this dynamic, rhetoric plays a powerful part in determining what is most fashionable. Rhetoric can be very persuasive and so texts (fashionable models) ascend and descend depending on which wins, often momentarily, the challenge for power and dominance. Knowledge and power become inseparable in epistemological and discourse paradigms, as well as authoritative, underpinning normative and consensus approaches. When, then, does rhetoric become ideology and therefore more covert and subtle (that is, a deliberate attempt to mislead)? Paradigms contain epistemological assumptions which are the knowledge-creating practices which develop over time. To truly understand the effects of these on practice and how differing interpretations can be understood, it is, as Eco (1995) says, necessary to consult the truth tables.

Believability is central to acceptance of the WHO HFA and evaluation models and intertextuality would indicate that it is the interplay between the texts of the professional discipline, practice, research and political and economic texts of the time which can be problematic. If political ideology

MEDICAL

Evaluation is grounded in the principles of positivist methodology
It is quantitative
It is about measurement
It asks:

can it work?
does it work?
does it bring change?

PREVENTION

As in the medical model, it measures reductions in mortality and morbidity. A key question is 'do more people comply with the programme?'. It measures percentage increase in knowledge, awareness, change of attitude or knowledge and behaviour. Often uses indicators to collect data

EDUCATION

Evaluation is grounded in qualitative methodology and is referred to as PROCESS or ILLUMINATIVE EVALUATION. It seeks to give a complete picture of how and why an intervention worked or did not work. It too can use indicators as part of the process. Interviews or indepth case studies, action research may all be used

One way of beginning such a process in all preventive programmes or a cancer organization is to develop a systematic planned quality assurance programme

COMMUNITY DEVELOPMENT	POLITICAL RADICAL	EFFECTIVENESS
As in education or by combining medical prevention and education approaches by providing: • evidence of efficacy as a guide to planning programmes • process evaluation for collecting information throughout the implementation phase	This model promotes the use of all evaluation methodology. Integration. There is a distinction to be made between the role of the experimental methodologies such as the randomized control trial and process evaluation	Both experimental and process evaluation have distinct roles in evaluation research. The role of evidence-based trials is one to be funded nationally or regionally and the research should be ongoing, longitudinal and contribute to policy On a day-to-day basis (in reality) process evaluation gives credible data about the progress and development, success or otherwise of ongoing programmes. It too can contribute to the policy-making and decision-making process Practitioners and implementers cannot be expected to run RCTs; researchers can and their knowledge and results should be the starting point for practitioners. Once implemented, on a day-to-day basis, process evaluation illuminates why a programme is successful or unsuccessful and how it works in practice. Evaluation is about: • evidence-based trials which are ongoing providing epidemiological and effectiveness information for planning • formative evaluation as the starting point for practitioners; this includes needs assessment research and pilot testing of programmes • intermediate evaluation (at midpoint in programme cycle) • impact (short term) • summative (long-term action)

Figure 2.2 Thinking about evaluation. The models previously described help us to understand how the various professional disciplines select evaluation models. This figure illustrates the relationships between models of health and models of evaluation.

changes and becomes more dogmatic, either left or right leaning, the difference between persuasive rhetoric and ideology becomes blurred and dependent on the personalities who wield power. It can indeed become dangerous. Thus texts, particularly those which fall necessarily in the public domain by virtue of the fact that they require public money (tax), will be forced to change. This may change the nature of the discourse and thus health promotion and how it is carried out. Jingoism and derision play an important part in this by languaging the new world (grand plan, 'STORY'/ 'stories') into being and deriding the previous discourse and text (Chomsky, 1979, 1996; Pilger, 1986, 1992; Usher and Edwards, 1994). Silent texts, those used in the transformation of 'new' texts, are not always obvious or acknowledged. Rhetorical devices are used to produce a credible imitation, repeating previous versions now credited to those who transform the original.

As well as the dialectical argument there is a constant phenomenological dynamic (Scott's double hermeneutic – see Chapter 3) at work not only at the level of the ongoing interaction of the epistemological and the ontological but between texts and also between the theoretical and practice worlds, each influencing the other, as can be seen in Figure 2.3.

Depending on the interpretations of the epistemological and ontological, the political dialogue at particular historical points and who is interpreting the texts (the characters in the 'story/ies'), understanding of the nature and purpose of evaluation methodology/method may well vary. There is no one world of health promotion and no one way of promoting health or evaluating what it is we do. There are as many ways as there are texts, discourses and characters involved, all being influenced by the fashion of the time.

Logical positivism, justified as it is by foundationalism, seeks 'truth' and

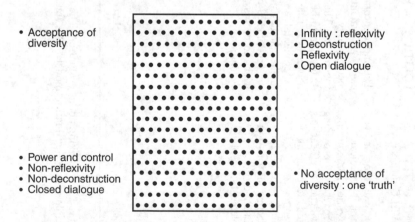

Figure 2.3 The phenomenological dynamic.

certainty. The qualitative approaches challenge this paradigm by intimating that evaluators interpret and understand 'meanings' (Weber's (1958) social action theories and Hammersley's (1992) theory of diversity) and the world of those researched. However, as Popper (1969) and Fox (1993) suggest, such 'certainty' and 'absolute truth' are evasive, constantly slipping from our grasp. Meanings too are problematic as the dynamic between the worlds described above is constantly changing in an interactive way. This suggests that it is necessary to work with similarity but also 'difference', to value difference as something which may indeed enrich this world of research/evaluation, using experience from all possible knowledge and practice fields to learn how we might know what it is we do and how we do it in this business of health promotion. This would suggest that there is an overconcern with rhetorical and ideological debates of a rational technical nature, which is really about power and knowledge which all too easily imitate the seeming 'ideal', empirical science (Spariosu, 1984). Health promoters/evaluators need to learn to value 'difference' to further inform policy and decision making and to ensure they have the best available information, judicial evidence (see Chapter 4). Usher would suggest that this can be achieved by reflexivity.

REFLEXIVITY AND THE RELATIONSHIP WITH IMPROVED PRACTICE IN EVALUATION OF INTERVENTIONS AND PROGRAMMES

As Usher and Edwards (1994) and Murdoch (1970) suggest, reflexivity is not just the understanding and conscious reporting of possible researcher/ practice bias. It goes far beyond this to an acceptance that researchers/ theoreticians/practitioners are creators of their texts and are therefore in and of them. They transform other texts, taken from a range of disciplines. Usher uses contextual analysis to illustrate the researcher autobiographical perspective but also the complex intertextuality which exists in most research and practice disciplines. The work of Propp (1968) and Silverman (1993) can be useful in analysing the 'STORIES/stories' which can be revealed by charting the history, characters and discourse in relation to the WHO consensus, HFA. These can be seen in Table 2.1. Usher's work can be helpful in understanding how powerful a tool reflexivity can be in health promotion and therefore emphasizes the need to be vigilant in understanding what health promotion is about; this can be seen in Tables 2.2 and 2.3 and Figure 2.4. By reading the texts in depth and carrying out a discourse analysis, the spheres of action can be illuminated. There is currently one 'grand plan' ('STORY') e.g. WHO/HFA but many 'stories' (ways of interpreting WHO/HFA), that is, ways of theorizing, researching and practising the implementation of such.

Table 2.1 Spheres of action (Weston, 1997). Reproduced with the permission of the University of Southampton.

Paradigm	*Sphere 1*	*Sphere 2*	*Sphere 3*	*Sphere 4*
Empiricist	Principles of WHO HFA (the 'STORY')	Positive healthy lifestyle change a 'story'	Individual behaviour change a 'story'	Self-efficacy a 'story'
Qualitative Educational/community	Principles of WHO HFA the 'STORY'	Positive health and lifestyle change a 'story'	Individual behaviour change Social and policy change a 'story'	Empowerment Avoidance of victim blaming a 'story'
Radical/political	Social and structural change Political action 'A STORY'	Health policy a 'story'	Equity, justice, human rights a 'story'	No Victim blaming a 'story'

Table 2.2 Reflexivity from the researcher point of view (Weston, 1997). Reproduced with the permission of the University of Southampton.

Paradigm	Context	Pre-text	Sub-text	Inter-text
Medical Empiricist	Biography – situated in the Qualitative paradigm. Female. Anti-authority	Resistant to this text because of its empirical roots – its authoritarian stance, its view of people as passive, its power	It goes against my beliefs about human beings, educational principles, my lack of confidence in mathematical statistics	This model intertextually plays with some things the researcher has feared as well as a lack of confidence with medical persona
Qualitative Education/community	Situated here and dominated by this in the past. Humanist beliefs	Resistant to any 'false' pretensions, false ways of promoting health. Feel health promotion is digging its own grave	My belief in the lack of need to have power relationships at all. Anarchic to some extent	My own biographical texts play very much with the anarchic political discourses, the humanist discourse, socialist political discourse and basic belief in human rights for all
Radical	This could be the same as the first, that is, medical paradigm. This is where I would like to be and like health promotion to be. Sometimes I do not have the confidence and courage to promote it	For me, this is the polarized position with the medical discourse, even though I know it is not so polarized. It is 'me' challenging systems which have bound me in the past	It definitely shows up my power, knowledge formation; the dislike of exclusive discourses, the snobbery and power they give people	Plays with my biography, my social class, my gender and my wish to work with equality, justice and human rights. No inscriptions

Table 2.3 Reflexivity: textual analysis from the paradigmatic perspective (Weston, 1997). Reproduced with the permission of the University of Southampton.

Paradigm	Context	Pretext	Subtext	Intertext
Empiricist	Researchers are trained in the experimental science and believe that there is 'a truth' Usually viewed as rational and grounded in patriarchal systems	Language, rational male dominated, discourse closed, embedded in rational science No grey areas	Power-knowledge embedded in pure science objectivity Medical scientific	Medicine, science, philosophy, politics, economics Top down, bottom up
Qualitative	Researchers are usually trained in education or social sciences, both male and female but suspect more female Some researchers from the empiricist school Many truths	Language 'woolly', neither one thing nor another. Purports to be on the 'people's side' but is not always. Embedded in sociology/ethnography, grey areas	Power-knowledge embedded in subjectivity, representation of the world Sociological/humanist	As above Interplay of some political historical literary texts, partnerships and democracy
Radical	Researchers could be from either of above. This is usually political, strong and definite views about: • society • people/individuals • rights • advocacy Could be either right or left politics	Language strong and dominant, black and white, no grey areas 'One truth' embedded in political discourses	Power-knowledge embedded in political discourses, right and left, as anti-everything Anarchic, but can also change things by rightness and justice	Politics, economics, human rights, history, the people and their needs Bottom up, top down

Empiricist	Research	Qualitative
Medical Prevention Protection Effectiveness	Evaluation	Education/radical Including action and developmental research Ethnography
RCT Experimental Quality assurance indicators		Process Illuminative Quality assurance/indicators

Figure 2.4 Intertextuality: research and evaluation paradigms (Weston, 1997). Reproduced with the permission of the University of Southampton.

By carrying out this exercise on the key leaders (characters) in the field and their texts, it is possible to identify their stance in relation to the texts they have relied upon and transformed, as well as the transformation.

By linking the key characters with Tables 2.1, 2.2 and 2.3, their theoretical and paradigmatic stance is illuminated. By combining with Table 2.1 it is possible to see how this researcher has interpreted and transformed their texts (that of the characters) in turn. This research needed to go a stage further if it was to claim that these interpretations are accurate. The author did, however, interview some of the key leaders in the field in the course of the research study but does not claim that her interpretation is 'true' or that the characters would necessarily agree with it. This analysis illustrates how important it is to be clear about:

- how the world of health promotion is interpreted (epistemological);
- what is done in this world (the ontological);
- appropriate evaluation strategies for such work rather than researcher-driven evaluation strategies. Arguably this may support the EU view that 'evaluation is an art, not a science'.

How these aspects are interpreted in the first instance, by the key characters and by this author who has then transformed their work, necessarily affects the interpretations underpinning this chapter.

EVALUATION AS AN ART: CONSENSUS ARGUMENTS

The EU has suggested that 'evaluation is an art, not a science' and as such, requires much careful planning and management. In an attempt to apply this to health promotion, it is necessary first to describe the parameters of the debate. Evaluation presents a methodological research and political dilemma. Over the last 30 years evaluation has become a separate field of enquiry, designed to illuminate why projects/programme/interventions are successful or not. A number of methods of teaching the ethical and political issues embedded in evaluation practice have been developed (Simons, 1987). It is political, having consequences both for those evaluated and those who are affected by it. This is often referred to as the macro and micro aspect of evaluation. Macro-level evaluation is that expected by funding bodies, planners and policy-makers and micro-level by those who have managed and developed the projects/programmes and who are therefore illuminated and questioned/interrogated. As Simons (1995) suggests, it is not just a technical exercise but a formal, systematic one. Public evaluation is still a relatively new field of enquiry, a little over 25 years old.

Texts on evaluation can be read in numerous ways, depending on who created the text and on who is reading and interpreting it. As Tones and Tilford (1994) suggest, even at the level of methodological debate, there is still no real consensus about methodology or agreement that evaluation is a research activity. Evaluation as a field has developed quickly and in educational evaluation, this led to the 'boomtown' concept described by Cronbach (1963, 1980).

However, for the purposes of this text there is an acceptance that most fields of practice have agreed that evaluation is an essential component of all programmes and actions (activities), that it is a research activity although not necessarily in the logical positivist /rational technical paradigm. On the issue of methodology, there is evidence of a growing consensus that programmes should be based on judicial evidence (in the ideal world) and that process evaluation is essential throughout the implementation phase. There is also consensus that judicial evidence or quantitative data are not useful without such a process evaluation. Developing a quality assurance programme should be a priority for organizations and for all their programmes and projects (Chemlinsky, 1994; van Driel et al., 1994).

The models of evaluation can be superimposed on those of research and the models of health, an example of intertextuality, as can be seen in Tables 2.2 and 2.3, but this also reveals imitative development as well as emerging narrative development: similarity giving way to difference.

The discourse on evaluation develops from that of the research paradigm in which it is grounded. Simons (1987), however, suggests that evaluation activities resemble policy and strategy research and therefore require lateral thinking and a range of research methodologies. Many evaluators see the benefit of a combination of methods referred to as methodological pluralism (House, 1981, 1993; Cronbach, 1980; Nutbeam, 1990; Steckler et al., 1992; Tones and Tilford, 1994; Baum, 1995). These various creators of texts are from different paradigmatic backgrounds – educational, political and public health – and so it would seem that the polarities and dualities are not as evident as at first thought (Steckler et al., 1992; Baum, 1995).

HISTORICAL PERSPECTIVES

Each discipline has developed its own evaluation discourse, exhausting the theory and the debate at particular times. There is only so much that can be done with a theoretical field. By studying the following fields and carrying out a comprehensive literature search, similar patterns have been revealed in the historical development of evaluation and research. The fields reviewed were:

- education;
- medicine;
- social services;
- EU structural projects;
- health service;
- business and commercial worlds.

These all use the same basic theory and practice and are all concerned with the same methodological debates. All interpret theory and practice differently in relation to the contexts in which they research or work.

METHODOLOGICAL DEBATE IN PUBLIC HEALTH

The debate revolves around whether accountability and effectiveness studies have more credibility than illuminative or process studies, imitative of Platonic, Socratic and Rousseau-esque 'ideals' (Spariosu, 1984). This can be summed up as whether measurement is more important than knowing whether a programme, project or organization is effective, that it works and gives value for money. According to the current debate, the challenge by the effectiveness movement has ensured that it is now in the dominant position, as empiricist models move into the ascendency. Yet the ongoing debate creates another space where process evaluation can re-enter as strategic shifts allow for continuous challenge. As can be seen from the earlier discourse analysis, such challenges are ongoing. Each of the fields studied had similar histories and Simons (1987) sums up this historical development cogently in her own text. Her text was validated by studying the EC Task Force documents and the work of other authors (Cronbach, 1963, 1980; Scriven, 1967; Stake, 1967; Cochrane, 1972; Guba and Lincoln, 1976; House, 1980, 1981, 1993; McDonald and Roe, 1984; Baric, 1986; Sanson-Fisher, 1985, etc.; Parlett and Hamilton, 1987; Majaro, 1988; Kok and de Vries, 1989; Nutbeam, 1990; Green and Kreuter, 1991; Hawe *et al.*, 1993; Russell, 1993; Tones and Tilford, 1994; Chalmers and Altman, 1994). This was supported by the systematic review carried out for the EU Cancer Programme (Weston, 1997), the published papers on evaluation, the analysis of the randomized control trial and the qualitative studies analysed as well as the interviews with key leaders in the field.

In summary, the following patterns and similar discourses were revealed. The familiar arguments over historic periods of time have been:

- cost effectiveness and measurement in many disciplines. For example, in education the numbers passing the 11+, truants, absenteeism, teacher statistics and now league tables and standards;
- epidemiology, mortality and morbidity statistics, in social services case numbers and problems linked to decision making and budgets for state benefit and, in the last few years, a return to these as important;
- accountability in terms of profit, saving of resources, scarce resource arguments;
- epidemiology, bed use, training, infection rates and so on and now a competitive league table for waiting lists, prevention of chronic disease through lifestyle behaviour change which, of course, is dominantly individual and without recognition of poverty and social contexts as well as health policy (HEA, 1997).

It was not until the late 1960s and early 1970s that a systematic formal curriculum evaluation in the USA and the UK was developed and evaluation theory entered the debate. At the same time in the business world there was much debate about improving the working of organizations in order to enhance their performance. Issues of quality assurance came onto the scene. Most practitioners think this innovation came from Japan but in fact it began in the USA and the Japanese imported it (Majaro, 1988). Cronbach (1963) articulated the need for providing information on decision-making in educational theory. Scriven (1967) created terminology such as formative and summative evaluation and Stake (1967) suggested broadening the base of evaluation data to include information on process to enable judgements about policy and planning, each transforming the narrative.

The framework for these evaluations, in this historical context, was objectives led. It concentrated on the planning process, using experimental research (pre-test/post-test in the main), systems analysis and cost effectiveness. In health and medicine this was mirrored by the use of the clinical trial, with the randomized control trial as the primary method being promoted for judicial evidence in the current climate. However, these methods were seen as inadequate to analyse and understand complex phenomena and educational/social programmes (Pirie et al., 1994). Development from this point became more pragmatic and more grounded in the qualitative.

The main protagonists for change in education were McDonald and Roe (1984) and Parlett and Hamilton (1987) who both influenced the health promotion field with the notion of illuminative evaluation. This transgressed the experimental models of the previous two decades. It has to be remembered, too, that much educational measurement had been found wanting and in some cases such quantification bias had forced education into a crisis. It is interesting that this has come full circle and the modern trend is a reversion to quantification in terms of league tables, reducing waiting lists, reducing the numbers on benefit and, in the business world, downsizing. The human and social elements in this equation are once again forgotten. As health promotion evolved, the time was ripe for change. This applied to social services, to the health service and to health promotion too. These services were undergoing change. If intertextuality with political texts is taken into account, then change and the ascendency of a new discourse, process or illuminative, was closely linked with left-wing political change throughout Europe, postwar euphoria and the cold war. This was based on the notion that there was a better world, a better way to do things than in the past. So the empiricist paradigm for evaluation was in decline, with the demise of 'a grand plan', and the qualitative became dominant. With the new paradigm came new methods: case studies, ethnographic studies, social anthropological studies, action research and developmental studies. Practitioners used qualitative methods, grounded in the phenomenological to collect data, as opposed to quantitative in the empiricist paradigm.

The next phase of development concerned the political decision-making process, the informing and development of policy and strategy. House (1981) suggested that evaluation is an integral part of the political processes of society. The debates still centred around methodology overshadowing the political issues, such as power, and there was much questioning about how evaluators give or take power depending on the stakeholders who required the evaluation and those to be evaluated. These were and still are very important aspects of the evaluation process. Evaluation can mean more resources or fewer resources, the difference between a programme (or job) surviving and not. House (1980) and Simons (1987) suggest that if evaluation was to be democratic, it was important to ask the following questions for every evaluation:

- What is the purpose of evaluation?
- Who should do it and what methods should be used?
- Who are the audiences, who will have the results and in what form?
- Who are the major stakeholders and what are their needs?

These need to be explicit for the planning stage (see Chapter 6) so all parties know where they are. To bring this up to date, there does seem to be general consensus on these aspects today.

Evaluation is political, the programmes are creations of political decisions; evaluation feeds into this political process and evaluation always has a political stance. By looking at intertextuality, it becomes apparent that there has been a shift in the discourse and perhaps even in the 'grand plan' in evaluation during the late 1980s and 1990s. The political texts have moved to the conservative right and accountability and measurement have been reborn, re-invented and transformed. This in turn has once again refocused a rather polarized debate on methodology and it could be argued that it has taken health full circle back to a medical paradigm and thus to some derision of the community and education models. This reading points to the medical/scientific model currently being in the ascendency in health promotion. It is the Parlett and Hamilton (1987) argument in reverse.

ETHICAL PARAMETERS

The ethical arguments (see Chapter 9) have also had a long history. Ethical theory has been used to both sell and justify evaluation and the various methods. However, there is a need, accepted by almost all the authors, for democratic and ethical parameters to be agreed by all parties (stakeholders) in any evaluation research protocol. These apply to the concepts of fairness and justice for all stakeholders and need to be agreed by discussion between all partners. It is particularly important to distinguish between judgements based on the data collected and subjective assessment of such data. Currently, suggests Simons (1995), there is a need to be aware that the climate in which evaluations take place has changed and is still changing. It can be a political nightmare. Evaluators need very clear guidelines for their work, whether in-house or as independent external evaluators. They must remain independent but of course they are not autonomous. A further dimension is in the designing of research protocols and interpretation of results. Scott argues that it is most important that researchers are aware and reflexive about evaluation research. It is important to understand that paradigmatic arguments which serve to justify methodology may themselves mean that the research is unethicist, particularly in the possible manipulation of variables in the empiricist models but also in methodological terms in the design of the study. This can apply to both empirical and qualitative methodology. Researchers should not deceive themselves otherwise and need to be conscious of the effects of the research on all parties, as well as how they too construct the social world through both their research and value systems.

So, the current theory and practice of evaluation in respect of health promotion can be summed up in Figure 2.5.

The consensus on evaluation which can be gained from this literature search is that 'Evaluation is an art, not a science'. As an art form it requires:

Organize yourselves first: logistical steps
1. Set up a monitoring committee or a steering/management group
2. Appoint a neutral chairperson
3. Set up a timetable and venue of meetings
4. Decide working practices
5. Develop programme objectives closely linked to EC core programme objectives

Remember the seven steps of the evaluation process
1. Set up a monitoring committee which has overall responsibility
2. Set up an evaluation steering group to take on the day-to-day management of evaluation
3. Agree to evaluation questions through open discussion and the type of evaluation necessary. These should be directly linked to programme objectives
4. Write the contracts and tenders
5. Make a time plan/work plan or gannt chart as a guide to working practice
6. Choose evaluators and obtain justification of the methodology they intend to use. This must link with the objectives and evaluation questions
7. Consider the dissemination process, particularly of the evaluation report. You may need different reports for different audiences

Figure 2.5   The logistical steps of evaluation using cancer as example.

- planning;
- a methodological framework which is appropriate for answering the questions set. These should be related to the outcome objectives for the programme;
- an active partnership of all stakeholders from the early stages;
- contracts agreed by all parties;
- evaluators, appointed by an agreed process;
- the interviewing of prospective evaluators during which they should be able to justify their methodology;
- agreement by all parties about the dissemination process, agreed at the early planning stages.

The style of reports is also important and there should be agreement about this and what kind of information is required, what data are necessary and how the results will best influence practice. Evaluation is a policy issue and organizations require a policy about it. This places it in the category of a developing narrative and an open debate. It is not a mere imitation or repetition of the empirical models, especially the clinical trial.

REFERENCES

Baric, L. (1986) The singer and the song. *Journal of the Institute of Health Education*, **33**, 124–129.

Baum, F. (1995) Researching public health behind the qualitative–quantitative methodological debate. *Social Science and Medicine*, **40**(4), 459–468.

Blair, T. (1997) Election address, BBC TV, May.

Chalmers, I. and Altman, D. (1995) *Systematic Reviews*, London: BMJ Books.

Chemlinsky, E. (1994) *Where we stand today in the practice of evaluation: some reflections*. Paper given to First Conference of European Evaluation Society, The Hague, December.

Chomsky, N. (1979) Language and responsibility. In B. Magee (ed.), *Men of Ideas*, Oxford: Oxford University Press.

Chomsky, N. (1996) Politics. In *The New Statesman*, August.

Cochrane, A.L. (1972) *Effectiveness and Efficiency: Random Reflections on the Health Service*, Cambridge: Memoir Club.

Cronbach, L.J. (1963) Course improvement through evaluation. *Teachers College Record*, **64**, 672–683.

Cronbach, L.J. (1980) *Towards Reform of Program Evaluation*, New Jersey: Jossey Bass.

Eco, U. (1995) *Six Walks in the Fictional Woods*, London: Harvard University Press.

Evans, D., Head, M.J. and Speller, V. (1994) *Assuring Quality in Health Promotion: How to Develop Standards of Good Practice*, London: HEA.

Fox, N.J. (1993) *Postmodernism, Sociology and Health*, Milton Keynes: Open University Press.

Giddens, A. (1991) *Modernity and Self-identity: Self and Society in the Late Modern Age*, Cambridge: Polity Press.

Green, L.W. and Kreuter, M.W. (1991) *Health Education Planning: An Educational and Environmental Approach*, Palo Alto, CA: Mayfield.

Guba, E. and Lincoln, Y. (1976) *Effective Evaluation* New Jersey: Jossey Bass.

Hammersley, M. (1992) *What is wrong with Ethnography?* London: Routledge.

Hawe, P., Degeling, D. and Hall, J. (1993) *Evaluating Health Promotion*, Sydney: Maclennan and Petty.

Health Education Authority (1997) *Inequalities in Health: Insights from the Qualitative Research Literature*, London: HEA.

House, E.G. (1981) *Evaluating with Validity*, Beverly Hills: Sage.

House, E.G. (1993) *Professional Evaluation: Social Impact and Political Consequences*, London: Sage.

Kok, G. and De Vries, H. (1989) *Primary Prevention of Cancers – The Need for Health Education and Intersectoral Health Promotion in Reducing the Risk of Cancer*, Milton Keynes: Open University Press.

McDonald, R. and Roe, E. (1984) *Informed Professional Judgement: A Guide to Evaluation in Post Secondary Education*, London: BPS Books.

Majaro, S. (1988) *The Creative Gap. Managing Ideas for Profit*, Guildford: Longman.

MEANS, EU (1995) *Methods for Evaluating Actions of Structural Nature*, Brussels: EC Centre for Evaluation Expertise.

Minkler, M. (1994) Ten commitments for community health education. *Health Education Research*, **9**(4), 527–534.

Murdoch, I. (1970) *The Sovereignty of Good*, Oxford: Oxford University Press.

Nutbeam, D. (1990) Evaluation in health education: a review of possibilities and problems. *Journal of Epidemiology and Community Health*, **44**(2), 83–89.

Parlett, M. and Hamilton, D. (1987) Evaluation as illumination: a new approach to the study of innovatory programmes. In R. Murphy and H. Torrance (eds) *Evaluating Education: Issues and Methods*, London: PCP Education Series.

Pilger, J. (1986) *Heroes*, Reading: Vintage.

Pilger, J. (1992) *Distant Voices*, Reading: Vintage.

Pirie, P.L., Stone, E.J., Assal, A.R., Flora, J.A. and Baschewsky-Schneider, U. (1994) Programme evaluation: strategies for community-based health promotion programmes: perspectives from cardiovascular disease community research and demonstration studies. *Health Education Research Theory and Practice*, **9**(1), 23–36.

Popper, K. (1959) *The Logic of Scientific Discovery*, New York: Basic Books.

Popper, K. (1969) *Conjecture and Refutation*, London: Routledge and Kegan Paul.

Propp, V. (1968) *The Morphology of the Folk Tale*, 2nd edn, Austin, TX: University of Texas.

Russell, I. & NHS Wales Office of Research and Development and University of Wales (1993) *Towards a Knowledge-based Health Service*, Cardiff: NHS.

Sanson-Fisher, R.W. (1985) Commentary: behavioural science and its relation to medicine – a need for positive action. *Community Health Studies*, **IX**(3), 275–283.

Sanson-Fisher, R.W. (1991) *Some mechanisms for encouraging behaviourally orientated cancer research in Australia*, Newcastle, NSW: University of Newcastle.

Sanson-Fisher, R.W. (1993a) Primary and secondary prevention of cancer: opportunities for behavioural scientists. In S. Maes, H. Leventhal and M. Johnston (eds) *International Review of Health Psychology, Vol 2*, Chichester: John Wiley.

Sanson-Fisher, R.W. (1993b) *Achieving Cancer Control through Behavioural Change, An Overview/Report*, Wallsend, NSW: New South Wales Cancer Council Cancer Education Research Project.

Sanson-Fisher, R.W. and Redman, S. (1986) The challenge of community health. In *Health Care: Behavioural Approach*, Grune and Stratton.

Sanson-Fisher, R.W. and Byles, J. (1990) The role of health social science in preventive medicine. In J. McNeil, R. King, G. Jennings and J. Powles (eds) *A Textbook of Preventive Medicine*, Melbourne: Edward Arnold.

Sanson-Fisher, R.W. and Turnbull, D. (1993) *To Do or Not to Do? Ethical Problems for Behavioural Medicine*, Newcastle, NSW: University of Newcastle.

Sanson-Fisher, R.W. and Campbell, E. (1994) Health research in Australia – its role in achieving the goals and targets. *Health Promotion Journal of Australia*, **4**(3), 28–33.

Sanson-Fisher, R.W., Schofield, M.J. and Girgis, A. (1992) Why is there a need for behavioural research in cancer control? *Journal of Cancer Care*, **1**, 113–123.

Sanson-Fisher, R.W., Girgis, A., Redman, S. and Schofield, M.J. (1993) *The Staged Approach to Health Promotion Practice and Research: an Overview*, Wallsend, NSW: New South Wales Cancer Council Cancer Education Research Project.

Scriven, M. (1967) The methodology of evaluation. In American Educational

Research Association, *Perspectives of Curriculum Evaluation*, Chicago: Rand McNally.

Silverman, D. (1993) *Interpreting Qualitative Data Methods for Analysing Talk and Interaction*, Milton Keynes: Open University Press.

Simons, H. (1987) *Getting to Know Schools in a Democracy: The Politics and Process of Evaluation*, Lewes: Falmer Press.

Simons, H. (1995) Class notes, MPhil/PhD, University of Southampton, UK.

Spariosu, M. (1984) *Mimesis in Contemporary Theory, Volume 1. The Literary and Philosophical Debate*, Philadelphia: John Benjamins Publishing Company.

Stake, R.E. (1967) *The countenance of educational evaluation. Teachers College Record*, **68**(7), 235–240.

Steckler, A. et al (1992) Towards integrating qualitative and quantitative methods: an introduction. *Health Education Quarterly*, **19**(1), 1–8.

Tones, K. and Tilford, S. (1994) *Health Education, Effectiveness, Efficiency and Equity*, 2nd edition, London: Chapman and Hall.

Usher, R. and Edwards, R. (1994) *Post Modernism and Education: Different Voices, Different Worlds*, London: Routledge.

Van Driel, G.W., Keijsers, J.F.E. and Molleman, G.R. (1994) *Effectiveness of Health Education/Health Promotion: From Research Analysis to Guidelines for Practitioners*, Utrecht: Dutch Centre for Health Promotion and Education.

Weber, M. (1958) in *Sociology: Themes and Perspectives*, M. Haralambos (1980) (ed.), Trowbridge: UTP.

Weston, R. (1997) *The myth-makers in health promotion: is the randomised control trial the gold standard?* PhD Thesis, University of Southampton, UK.

World Health Organization (1946) *Constitution*, Geneva: WHO.

World Health Organization (1978) *Report on The Conference on Primary Health Care*, Alma Ata, 6–12 September, Geneva: WHO.

World Health Organization (1984) *Health Promotion: A Discussion Document on the Concepts and Principles*, Copenhagen: WHO Regional Office for Europe.

World Health Organization (1985) *Targets for Health For All*, Copenhagen: WHO Regional Office for Europe.

World Health Organization (1986) *Ottawa Charter for Health Promotion*, An International Conference on Health Promotion, 17–21 November, Copenhagen: WHO Regional Office for Europe.

World Health Organization (1992) *Health Dimensions of Economic Reform*, Geneva: WHO.

Qualitative approaches to evaluations of health-promoting activities

3

David Scott

The purposes of evaluation in health promotion are much contested. Herman *et al.* (1987) identify seven models. The first is goal-orientated evaluation (cf. Bloom *et al.*, 1971), in which an assessment is made of the efficiency, effectiveness and economy of an intervention, where efficiency is defined as the degree to which the programme has achieved its aims and objectives; effectiveness is whether the objectives of the programme have led to desired outcomes; and economy is whether those outcomes have been achieved economically (Naidoo and Wills, 1994).[1] The second is decision-orientated evaluation (cf. Stufflebeam *et al.*, 1971) in which evaluators strive to improve the judgements made by policymakers. The third is evaluation research (cf. Campbell, 1972) where the focus is on explaining effects or outcomes and identifying their causes. The fourth is responsive evaluation where the evaluator's task is to provide descriptions of the process of the intervention and in particular of the value perspectives of participants (cf. Stake, 1967). The fifth model explicitly accepts the criticism levelled at goal-orientated evaluation and argues that evaluation should be goal-free, not in the sense that the values of the data collector do not influence the evaluation, but that the aims and objectives of the intervention as laid down by the project team may fail to give an adequate account of the process of the intervention (cf. Scriven, 1967). In contrast, Wolf (1975) suggests that evaluators should provide contrasting points of view to the accepted descriptions of what is taking place. Finally Patton's (1986) utilization-orientated evaluation model suggests that evaluators should act to maximize the way findings can be used by different stakeholders.

Each of these models concentrates on different aspects of the evaluation process. In particular, they take different positions as to whether evaluation of health promotion initiatives should concentrate on processes or products; on whether interventions should be evaluated in terms of original intentions or as goal free; and on which stakeholders' (policymakers, programme constructors, participants) interests should be of prime concern. Finally, there is disagreement about whether evaluators of health promotion activities should aim to produce generalizable knowledge or understandings of particular processes; in short, whether evaluation should be formative and particularistic or summative and generalizable.[2]

This chapter will consider the nature of evaluation, examine the relationship between evaluation and research, contrast different methodological frameworks and methods and examine different rationales for evaluating health-promoting activities. It will therefore seek to address philosophical issues and suggest that evaluators have to ask themselves questions about the methods they use and, more importantly, the relationship between those methods and the methodological frameworks which underpin them. This, by definition, focuses attention on epistemological and ontological concerns[3] and seeks to answer questions about the nature of the descriptions evaluators make about health promotion.

EVALUATION AND RESEARCH

Whether evaluation and research should be considered as separate activities has proved controversial, with some (cf. Simons, 1987; MacDonald, 1984) designating evaluation as a separate activity; and others (Norris, 1992; Tones and Tilford, 1994)[4] arguing that the division is simply one of emphasis. Glass and Worthen (1971) cite eleven factors which distinguish evaluation from research.

1. *The rationale for the enquiry* – research is pursued for disinterested reasons such as the production of knowledge, whereas evaluation is conducted to provide solutions to practical problems.
2. *The aims of the enquiry* – research is conducted in order to come to definite conclusions about reality; evaluation is designed to contribute to better decision making in practical situations.
3. *Laws as opposed to description* – research is nomothetic in orientation and thus seeks to make law-like statements about reality; evaluation is concerned to describe particular cases or events.
4. *The nature of explanation* – research always has to concern itself with why or how questions, such as whether the health promotion intervention will lead to a more healthy life; evaluation may simply concentrate on whether the expressed purposes of the evaluation have been achieved or not.

5. *Autonomy and control in the enquiry* – researchers have a greater freedom to set the boundaries of the enquiry, whereas evaluators always have to take into consideration the wishes of various stake-holders as to the shape and direction of the evaluation.

6. *Relation to social utility* – whereas research may indirectly contribute to contemporary policy debates, evaluation is directly concerned to do this.

7. *Scale of the enquiry* – research is concerned with large issues of social importance; evaluation concentrates on carefully delineated small-scale areas of social life.

8. *Interpenetration of values* – research offers value-free knowledge of social processes, whereas in evaluation, value issues are central.

9. *Methods of enquiry* – researchers in the quest for generalizable knowledge employ methods which fit with experimental and correlational designs, whereas evaluators are more concerned to use methods which fit with qualitative and ethnographic designs.

10. *Criteria for making judgements* – research is judged by traditional criteria such as sound internal validity, credible external validity, reliability and objectivity; evaluation, on the other hand, is judged by criteria such as credibility, transferability, dependability and confirmability (cf. Guba and Lincoln, 1985).

11. *Disciplinary focus* – researchers operate from within one disciplinary perspective, whereas evaluators are more likely to pursue their enquiries within a multidisciplinary perspective.

Before we discuss these, it is worth looking at another set of arguments that attempt to distinguish evaluation from research. It should be noted that this list points to differences of emphasis rather than clearcut distinctions. Smith (1982) suggests that evaluators: may be more concerned to assess the achievement of desirable goals; may be more constrained by the needs of stakeholders, in particular funders; may operate formatively; may have to negotiate between a variety of stakeholders with their own vested interests; may have less control over choice of research methods and methodology; may be more circumscribed by time constraints; and generally seek to influence decision-makers rather than provide generalizable knowledge about health promotion activities. This second list, by virtue of how it is constructed, has blurred the boundaries between research and evaluation.

The first list essentially locates the research process in a positivist framework; that is, objective reality can be grasped; researchers can remain neutral and bracket out their values from the process of enquiry; observations and generalizations are atemporal and asituational and enquiry is considered to be an objective activity (cf. Denzin, 1989). In other words, as Glass and Worthen (1971:153) understand research, it is an 'activity aimed at obtaining generalizable knowledge by contriving and testing claims about relationships amongst variables or describing generalizable phenomena'. Evaluation is therefore understood in opposition to this and as that activity which concerns itself with meaning, interpretive activity, localized and constrained situations, action perspectives and, furthermore, as inferior as a knowledge-producing activity. If research is understood in a different way, either as embracing interpretive perspectives or as replacing traditional notions of research, then the distinction between research and evaluation suggested by Glass and Worthen loses much of its force. Indeed, Smith (1982) implicitly acknowledges this since his list focuses on practical issues of conducting evaluations and in particular, how evaluators can collect useful data about health promotion interventions, given the inherent instability of such settings. As we have seen, such debates focus on purposes, rationales and relations with stakeholders, but above all on methodological frameworks. It is with the latter that we are now concerned.

POSITIVISM

The dominant and traditional model of evaluation is underpinned by a social theory known as positivism. However, it is difficult to say what it is. Kolakowski (1975) argues that a positivist conception of the world includes four elements: phenomenalism, nominalism, the separation of facts and values and the unity of the scientific method. Briefly, phenomenalism refers to the belief that as observers of the world we are only entitled to deal with phenomena as they appear to us and not to hidden or concealed essences. Natural and social scientists therefore deal with the relationships between these observed phenomena as they manifest themselves in regular patterns. The second element is nominalism. This is where the world is said to consist of objects which cannot be reduced in any way. In short, that we can discover facts about the world, which can then be used as building blocks in the development of theory. These facts exist by virtue of what the world is and do not depend in any way on their perception or cognition by social actors. This would seem to suggest that the relation between the world and our descriptions of it is unproblematic. Indeed, that a simple correspondence theory can be adduced to explain the relation, so that words and numbers are simply the means by which such phenomena are made intelligible.[5]

The third element is the separation of facts and values and logically follows from the nominalist doctrine discussed above. As Kolakowski (1975:13) argues: 'The phenomenalist, nominalist conception of science has another important consequence, namely, the rule that refuses to call value judgements and normative statements knowledge'. Logical positivists (cf. Ayer, 1936, amongst others) would go further and suggest that those branches of philosophy such as ethics and aesthetics which deal primarily with issues of judgement and value cannot legitimately be described as knowledge at all. Thus, ethical judgements are understood as emotive outbursts which cannot be evaluated as true or false. We may express value judgements about the world but we cannot expect them to be anything other than arbitrary choices and certainly they cannot qualify as scientific statements. The fourth element is the fundamental belief in the unity of the scientific method which is that there is only one correct way of understanding natural and social phenomena and that scientific detach-ment and objectivity constitute the right method.

These four principles lead to a view of knowledge which is concerned with the establishment of general laws or nomothetic statements about the world (both in its physical and social forms). These laws allow replicability of research, in that their discovery can be verified by other researchers who adopt similar procedures – those procedures or rules consist of public or verifiable criteria by which descriptions of the social world can be judged. These general laws consist of 'the constant conjunction of atomis-tic events or states of affairs, interpreted as the objects of actual or possi-ble experience' (Bhaskar, 1979:158).

A number of objections have been made to this way of understanding. The first is that data about the world are always informed by theoretical frameworks. The second objection follows from this and suggests that this implies a close relationship between knower and known which cannot be accommodated within a model of the disinterested observer of events. Thus at the very least this implies a reconceptualization of the notion of objectivity. It is important to understand that accepting this reconceptuali-zation and certainly weakening of the naive objectivist position does not imply that it is not possible to adopt a realist position.[6] What it does imply is that any realist position adopted has to take into consideration the inescapable limitations imposed on us by our locatedness in discourses, power plays, environments and time.

The third objection stems from the inability of social scientists to develop general laws and argues that because social life and, more particu-larly, the relationship between constructs developed by observers and those used by social actors are so arranged, then nomothetic descriptions of social life and educational activities are rarely possible. The double hermeneutic referred to above, with its two-way relationship between social actors' and social observers' interpretations, at best allows struc-tures or persistent relations to be only relatively enduring. Furthermore, the interpretive element involved in this means that we cannot take for granted that the categories we use to determine social facts are accurate unless we build into our research methodology a self-referential element.[7] As soon as we do this, we create open systems whereby we cannot be sure that the cases we have used to determine patterns of social life are in fact the same across time and place.

The fourth objection again follows from this. If it is difficult to imagine social laws being developed, then the predictive power of social descriptions is considerably weakened. Furthermore, unlike the natural sciences, any predictions we do make may influence the activities of those affected by them, thus changing their nature and at the same time decreasing our certainty about those predictions. The fifth objection is alluded to above and suggests that if we are only concerned with events and their constant conjunction, we are concerned merely with appearances and have ignored fundamental or underlying essences. Finally, an objection is made that the universalizing of method by which we can come to understand the world ignores the fact that method is both constitutive of the data we collect and immersed in specific and time-bound epistemological frameworks or, as Macintyre (1988) calls them, 'traditions of knowledge'.[8] Furthermore, understanding these 'traditions of knowledge' can only be attained from within; that is, in order to critique such frameworks, we can only do so from within the traditions of thought which sustain them.

PARADIGMATIC DEBATES

What this means is that research/evaluation cannot be treated as a pragmatic activity and that, as a result, researchers/evaluators need to answer philosophical, in particular epistemological, questions such as: What is the proper relationship between the evaluator and evaluatees? How can we know reality? What is it? etc. Researchers therefore, knowingly or not, are always located within methodological frameworks which implicitly answer some of the questions posed above. Denzin and Lincoln (1995) suggest that there are four different ways of conceptualizing this debate. The first is where those criteria used to judge natural scientific work are thought equally appropriate for the study of the social world. (This is an a-paradigmatic perspective.) The second position is opposed to this since the argument is that the social and natural worlds are qualitatively different and thus different criteria are appropriate for making judgements about each. (This is a di-paradigmatic perspective.) The third position is that there are no appropriate criteria for the study of the social world. (This is a multiparadigmatic perspective.) Finally, there is a fourth position which is that new criteria need to be developed which are appropriate for all forms of research but which explicitly involve a rejection of the assumptions which underpin positivism. (This is a uni-paradigmatic perspective.[9])

These debates are not just esoteric, but have real and material effects on the business of evaluation and research. This is because, depending on the position taken by the evaluator in terms of their paradigmatic perspective, they will adopt different positions on some of the important questions that need to be answered. Contra Bryman (1988), researchers/evaluators are confronted by a number of dilemmas in the field which cannot be solved pragmatically, but only by reference to epistemological and ontological perspectives. Bryman (1988:125) argues that fieldwork is a social activity and thus appropriate fieldwork behaviour cannot be ethically or normatively orientated, but is fundamentally a pragmatic affair: 'The problem with the "ought" view is that it fails to recognize that a whole cluster of considerations are likely to impinge on decisions about methods of data collection'. In a sense, this viewpoint acknowledges its own flaw, which is that it conflates normative and descriptive accounts of research. That evaluators in the past have paid scant attention to epistemological and ontological concerns is no guide as to how they should have behaved or should behave in the future.

THE QUALITATIVE/QUANTITATIVE DIVIDE

The most profound divide is between qualitative and quantitative researchers. The two main forms of quantitative research are experimental (or quasi-experimental where it is not possible to choose randomly groups or individuals for comparative purposes) and correlational. Each of these is problematic. Experimental researchers have been criticized on a number of grounds. In essence, these criticisms are threefold. First, many things are not easy to test for. Effects may be more subtle or difficult to conceptualize than experiment allows for. This point is particularly relevant to the time dimension of experiments, since effects of interventions are deemed to show up either partially or completely at certain definite moments of time which the experimenter is able to identify and thus appropriate as testing moments. Second, the experimental researcher studies human interaction in artificial settings and as a result it may be difficult to draw valid conclusions which relate to real-life situations; in other words, experiments may be ecologically invalid. Third, experimenters may not be able to capture the culture of the setting being investigated, operating as they do by reducing aspects of social life to sets of variables which, for the purposes of producing mathematical models, they then operationalize by reducing complex human activities to numbers. Indeed, critics (Giddens, 1984, and others) would go further and suggest that social phenomena cannot be properly understood without referring to the explanations given by social actors for their behaviours and activities. This last point refers to experimental or correlational research.

Two further issues need to be addressed. The first concerns the implicit unilinear model of causation subscribed to by correlational researchers. Health education practice may be conceived as deliberative action designed to achieve certain ends. What this implies is that there may be a number of different ways which are equally appropriate to achieve those ends. Indeed, participants in health promotion interventions may respond in different ways to different initiatives. However, the use of mathematical models to describe health education settings and the production of prescribed lists of specified behaviours would suggest a unilinear approach to health promotion. Quantitative modelling necessarily leads to certain ways of understanding health promotion settings and precludes others.

The second issue concerns the relationship between correlations and causal mechanisms. Even if a correlation can be established between two variables, it is still not possible to assert that the one caused the other to happen in an unproblematic way. There is always the possibility of a third variable causing variance in both. Furthermore, we cannot be sure as to which variable occurred first. Correlations are no more than the recording of relationships of variables or the constant conjunction of events. Realists such as Bhaskar (1989) reject the notion that these constant conjunctions of events necessarily represent reality. He talks about two different realms – the epistemological and the ontological. Causal mechanisms reside in the ontological realm, while constant conjunctions of events reside in the epistemological realm. The problem for evaluators of health promotion activities is to bridge the gap between the epistemological and the ontological, if it is understood that there is inevitably a gap between appearance and reality. Reality, as Bhaskar understands it, can be characterized in four ways: there are objective truths about the world whether we can know them or not; our knowledge of the world is always fallible because any claims we make about it can be disputed; there are transphenomenalist truths whereby we can only have knowledge of appearances and not necessarily of underlying structures or causal mechanisms; and even more importantly, there are counterphenomenalist truths in which those deep structures actually have misleading appearances, that is those appearances may be in conflict with the mechanisms that sustain them.

There are two consequences of this division between appearance and reality. First, the designation of correlations does not necessarily lead to the uncovering of causes. If we conflate the two, we are guilty of what Bhaskar calls the ontic fallacy, that is, the mixing up of epistemological and ontological phenomena. This is most obvious in some well-known examples. A hooter in London signalling the end of the day's work in a factory does not cause workers in Birmingham to pack up and go home, even if a correlation can be established between the two phenomena. A good correlation has been discovered between human and stork birth rates over a period of time in various regions of Sweden, but it is clear that the one does not cause the other to happen. Both these examples show what may be called spurious correlations in that the regularities so described do not relate in a straightforward manner to the causal mechanism which produced them. There may be two reasons for this. First, as we suggested above, a third variable may have acted on both to create the pattern we have observed. Second, as Bhaskar suggests, deep structures may have contradictory appearances. Evaluators of health promotion activities may therefore have to be extremely careful about ascribing causal relations to the observed constant conjunction of events. Furthermore, if this is correct, then there are two methodological solutions. The first is the use of experimental or quasi-experimental methods which I have discussed above. The second is qualitative or ethnographic approaches,[10] which form the subject matter of this chapter.

Meanwhile, we come to the other problem with mathematical models of health promotion activities and this is their ability to predict outcomes. If we uncover causal mechanisms and the claim is then made that these causal mechanisms apply in other circumstances, whether in place or time, then we are claiming that it is possible to develop laws about human activity, in a similar way to those laws developed by natural scientists. However, for us to be able to do this, we have to understand human beings in specific ways. First, that they are subject to laws of nature which compel them to behave in certain definite ways. Regardless of their complexity, the claim is made that if certain conditions are met, human beings will behave in certain predictable ways. As a result, it is possible for us to produce prescriptive lists of best possible practice in health promotion, confident as we are that if we set in motion the right health promotion intervention, it will have the desired effects. Second, that it is possible for us, given our locatedness in specific temporal and geographical localities to uncover those mechanisms. For Bhaskar, those mechanisms any way are only 'relatively enduring' and they are subject to decay because of the double hermeneutical nature of social reality and social research.

INTERPRETIVE PERSPECTIVES

Human beings both generate and are in turn influenced by social scientific descriptions of social processes. What this means is that any law-like statements we can make about health promotion activities are subject to evaluation and re-evaluation of their worth by practitioners acting subsequently. This re-evaluation means that those causal mechanisms inscribed in laws are suddenly no longer simple mechanisms which work on human beings, but now have added to them a further interpretive element. As Giddens (1984:31) argues, this 'introduces an instability into social research' which renders data and those findings produced by experimental or correlational methods problematic:

The social sciences operate with a double hermeneutic involving two-way ties with the actions and institutions of those they study. Socio-logical observers depend upon lay concepts to generate accurate descriptions of social processes; and agents regularly appropriate themes and concepts of social science within their behaviour, thus potentially changing its character. This ... inevitably takes it some distance from the 'cumulative and uncontested' model that natur-alistically-inclined sociologists have in mind.

This notion of the double hermeneutic points to a further sense we can give it. This is that human beings are reflexive and intentional actors who themselves are engaged in interpretive activity throughout their lives. However, evaluators themselves, in making interventions of whatever sort, are also themselves engaged in interpretive activity. Thus, we have a situa-tion (this is the act of doing research) in which evaluators are interpreting interpretations made by social actors. The nature of these interpretations is especially important in evaluation settings, constructed as they are in terms of unequal distributions of power and knowledge, vested interests and inadequate exchanges of information. This is so because the act of interpretation involves selection, the filtering out and organizing of a mass of data into a coherent pattern, which conforms to and has an effect on the way the evaluator already understands the world.

Giddens further argues that there are four levels of social research or evaluation. The first is the hermeneutical elucidation of the frame of meaning of the social actor(s) involved. The second is the investigation of context and the form of practical consciousness. The third is the identifica-tion of the bounds of knowledgeability and the fourth is the specification of institutional orders. His argument is that qualitative researchers either pay insufficient attention to the first or collect data about it in the wrong order or ignore it altogether. What this schema implies is that a purely phenomen-ological perspective is inadequate. This is so for four reasons: first, social actors operate within unacknowledged conditions, that is, societal struc-tures; second, there are unintended consequences of their actions; third, social actors operate through tacit knowledge which is hidden by virtue of what it is or, at least, cannot be and is not articulated during the formation of explanations of action; fourth, the social actor may be influenced by unconscious motivations. This points to the inevitable objectification involved in evaluation; that is, the going beyond the purely phenomenologi-cal perspective (cf. Bhaskar, 1989). However, as Giddens argues, this going beyond, in order for the explanation to be valid, has to involve an under-standing of the perspectives of social actors and the implication of this is that methods have to be appropriated which do not distort those meanings. There is therefore always an ethnographic moment in social research and this cannot legitimately be written out by quantitative researchers.

HEALTH PROMOTION MODELS

In terms of the evaluation of health promotion activities, this philosophical schema has certain consequences. What is being suggested is that those health promotion frameworks which evaluators subscribe to necessarily inform the collection of data and the design of their research. Tones and Tilford (1994:12) suggest the following three models, having provided the coda that these 'ideological constructions of reality' are in effect 'a simplified version of people's beliefs about the purposes of health education and the values loading those beliefs'. The first model is the medical or preventative model which aims to prevent and control disease by educating people, which in turn informs their attitudes and lifestyles and thus their health-promoting practices. The assumption being made is that knowledge of unhealthy practices will lead to social actors changing their lifestyle to prevent poor health in the future. This model is individualistic in its assumptions, functionalist in its view of human beings and ultimately reductionist in its stripping away to bare essentials the way human beings act.

The second framework has been appropriately entitled the radical model. Health and disease are now considered to result from social, cultural and environmental factors which can only be tackled at the level of the sociocultural. This model has been criticized for offering too deterministic a view of human behaviour. The debate between the two models discussed so far, the preventative and radical models, points to the central problem in social theory – that is, the dynamic which drives social life and to which evaluators need to pay careful attention. This is the debate between voluntarism and constraint or agency and structure. The radical model, on the surface, argues that structural constraints to healthy behaviour are such that health promotion activity has to be concentrated at the level of the sociopolitical. Inequalities of income contribute to unequal dietary provision so that one section of the community is more unhealthy than another. However, if we understand the relationship between agency and structure differently and as a dynamic and dialectical relationship, we perhaps can construct a model which takes full account of all the factors involved.

Giddens (1984), for instance, through his structuration approach, has attempted to reconcile agency and structure, so that human beings are neither the 'unwitting dupes' of structural forces beyond their control nor free unconstrained agents neither controlled nor influenced by those sets of relations and conjunctions which constitute society. For Giddens, actors continually draw on sets of 'rules and resources' which, once substantiated, allow social life to continue as they become routinized. Archer (1982:458) adopts a similar approach with her morphogenetic perspective, though she disputes the necessity of tying structure and agency so closely together: 'Structuration, by contrast, treats the ligatures binding structure, practice and system as indissoluble, hence the necessity of duality and the need to gain an indirect analytical purchase on the elements involved'. She also questions whether every human action, every facet of the particular human being, is involved in the ongoing moulding and remoulding of society that is implied by both structuration and morphogenetic cycles. She writes: 'There are a good many things about human beings and their doings (things biological, psychological and spiritual) which have a precious independence from society's moulding and may have little to do with re-modelling society' (1982: 455). Both Archer and Giddens argue that human beings play an active and intentional role in the construction of their world, though that building activity is always subject to structural constraints of various kinds. Human beings make their world in the context of previous attempts and at the same time transform those structures and change the conditions which influence subsequent moves to make the world. It is also important to recognize that whilst agency is responsible for structural transformation, in the process it simultaneously transforms itself (Archer, 1982).

In health promotion terms, human beings are able to make decisions about a health-promoting lifestyle but only within structural contexts – and these structural contexts provide good reasons as to why one decision is more rational than another. This meeting of agency and structure may be considered to be a third model or theoretical framework and has some affinities with empowerment models as they are described by Tones and Tilford (1990: 32): 'The term "empowerment" rather than "self-empowerment" has been deliberately selected in order to acknowledge the powerful effects of environmental factors in facilitating or hindering freedom of choice'. Let us reiterate the main principles of this approach. A healthy lifestyle involves both the adoption of healthy behaviours and the ability to make choices, even when there may be a tension between the two. However, the making of good choices always has to be understood as taking place within wider sociopolitical contexts, because it is these contexts which provide the social actor with good or bad reasons for behaving or not behaving in certain ways. Choosing between healthy and non-healthy options is always better informed by both knowledge of the effects of the desired behaviours and of the way the individual is positioned in society: in particular, the way that positioning relates to what Giddens (1984) has called "social markers" – that is, the gendered, racialized and classed nature of society. It is the prevailing discourses which surround such markers which allow some things to be said and others not to be. The implication of this is that an empowered individual is not just someone who makes the right decisions about a healthy lifestyle, but someone who has knowledge of the way society is organized and their place within these social arrangements. This also means that the acquiring of such knowledge about structural influences changes those structural influences, with the consequence that choice-making in the future is now circumscribed by a different set of arrangements.

Choice between these three models of health promotion, or these three ways of describing the purposes of health promotion, influences the amount and type of intellectual resources an evaluator brings to the setting or problem being evaluated. How the human being and human relations are understood determines the toolkit the evaluator uses during the evaluation. Furthermore, since we have characterized social life as a dynamic relationship between agency and structure or between voluntarism and constraint, the evaluation of health-promoting activities also needs to be understood as part of that dynamic process. In other words, the evaluator, by virtue of what they are doing, changes and intends to change what they are examining. For example, in process evaluation where the intention is to understand what has happened to an individual or group of individuals during a health promotion initiative, data are frequently collected by the evaluator about the beliefs and perceptions of social actors using interview techniques. Now, the interviewer, certainly when the interview is of the more unstructured kind, seeks to explore with the participant issues that are central to the project. This inevitably has the effect of increasing the knowledgeability of that participant as they are asked to reflect on their practices, lifestyle and ways of understanding the world, which in turn acts to both educate and empower them. The act of collecting data can never be a neutral descriptive procedure. It is not just that the health promotion initiative being evaluated seeks to change knowledge and attitudes, it is that the evaluation itself acts in a similar way. This applies regardless of the methodology used, whether it is experimental, correlational or phenomenological. This foregrounds the role of the evaluator and stresses the need for them to act reflexively and explicitly – that is, try to understand their role both as the collector of data and the expediter of a political project, in particular as these can be understood with regards to health.

REFLEXIVITY AND TEXTUALITY

This reflexive posture which the evaluator takes up has two elements. The first concerns the evaluator's role during the collection of data and the second concerns the text or evaluation report subsequently produced. In the first case, the evaluator, conscious of their immersion in a stratified social setting, seeks to understand both their own positioning and the way participants in their evaluation are located in relation to them. Interview data are therefore always the result of an asymmetrical relationship between interviewer and interviewee. The evaluator's concerns serve to structure the interviews and impose an agenda on them. Furthermore, the collection of interview data always involves a process of rationalization and this produces a gap between interviewees' accounts given in the course of an interview (or to a questionnaire) of how they behaved and what actually happened. This rationalizing process may be deliberate or unintended, distant or near in time to the activities being described and transparent or opaque. In the latter case, it allows many or few clues as to what really happened and employs or fails to employ rhetorical devices to protect its status as a definitive account. Interviewees may deliberately set out to deceive in order to protect their own interests, other interests or to place in the public domain an account of proceedings which they judge advances a particular political project more effectively (cf. Scott, 1996b). In evaluations of health promotion initiatives, this is particularly apposite, since evaluators frequently collect data about issues which respondents have cause to feel ashamed about (for example, cf. Cuckle and Vunakis, 1984).

The construction of the interview text involves complicated issues to do with the responsibilities of the interviewer towards those being interviewed and the degree of control which the interviewee is allowed. (Chapter 9 deals with the ethical and epistemological implications of this style of evaluation/research.) However, there is a second element of reflexivity and this concerns the textual nature of the evaluator's representations of reality. If, as I am suggesting, the evaluator needs to make explicit their value perspectives, the frameworks about health which they subscribe to and the context in which the data were collected to allow the reader purchase on and understanding of the nature of the conclusions which are drawn, then the way these matters are inscribed in the text is an important issue to consider. The traditional textual device is that of realism, in which the text is so constructed that it gives the impression that the inscription process is purely routine. Knowledge accrued by the evaluator represents unproblematically what has happened. Usher (1993) argues that the form a researched text generally takes is realist and representative, thus conveying the impression that it stands in some way for a set of phenomena that exist outside it and can be understood without reference to the way it was put together. If this fiction is to be exposed, then this demands a reflexive understanding of the evaluative experience. For Usher however, this does not mean that the evaluator simply has to supply a set of biographical facts to enable the reader to conceptualize the account they are reading. The reflexive posture is more fundamental:

> But the reflexive understanding which is always potentially present in doing research is not primarily the gaining of an awareness of one's own subjectivity, one's personality, temperament, values and standpoints. The desire that structures research is not the product of a

psychology which has been made "public" through honest introspection. Rather it is the effect of sociality and the inscription of self in social practices, languages and discourses which constitute the research process (Usher, 1993:9).

CONCLUSION

The argument developed in this chapter has four elements. First, in order for evaluators of health promotion activities to both make the correct decisions about the methods they use and understand their own procedures, they need to address fundamental epistemological and ontological questions. That is, they need to make explicit both to themselves and their readers what they are doing, what the nature of their findings is and what type of claims they are making in relation to health promotion. Second, because evaluators have to operate in the real world, they have to confront its multi-layered, power-infused and differentiated nature as they collect data. This means that data can never be collected in ideal circumstances (though this may represent an aspiration) and that as a consequence, there is always a gap between the perceptions of the investigator and what actually happened. The third part of the argument suggests a more profound difficulty, which is that evaluators represent, morally if not contractually, a number of different clients with different interests and different ways of understanding the world. This implies that evaluation is inevitably multi-perspectival and, furthermore, that those different perspectives may be in conflict.

The final part of the argument is that evaluators, however enlightened they may be, cannot operate as neutral collectors of data. Their activities affect in different ways the world they seek to describe. This again suggests that evaluation is always a political affair and that knowledge of health-promoting activities has to be understood as the development of new conceptions and perceptions of what a healthy society is. In short, we cannot as evaluators sustain the argument that our descriptions are not also prescriptions and that they are not underpinned by a set of frameworks about health, about the way we can come to know reality and about reality itself.

NOTES

1. These three terms, efficiency, effectiveness and economy, are not neutral descriptive terms but make reference to particular sets of values as they are used.
2. Though the terms formative and summative are generally used in the literature

to mean evaluation which takes place throughout the project and that which takes place at the end, they also indicate foci. Formative evaluation is particularistic and focused on the health promotion project being scrutinized; summative evaluation is more concerned with the production of generalizable knowledge which applies to larger populations than the one being investigated.

3. Epistemology refers to the way researchers and evaluators can come to know reality and thus is about knowing; ontology or being refers to the reality itself.

4. Tones and Tilford (1994: 50-51) make seven points in relation to this debate: research may have a wider range of purposes; may be less constrained by the needs of funders; is usually less concerned with immediate practical matters; may have to deal with less conflict because there are likely to be fewer stakeholders; may have greater control over choice of research methods; may be less concerned with time constraints; may be more concerned with the enhancement of understanding, as opposed to providing solutions to practical problems.

5. I have written about this elsewhere (Scott, 1996b). Macintyre (1988: 358) argues that relativist, perspectivist and rationalist positions all assume correspondence versions of our relations with reality. He suggests that: 'What is and was...highly misleading, was to conceive of a realm of facts independent of judgements or of any form of linguistic expression, so that judgements or statements could be paired off with facts, truth or falsity being the alleged relationship between such paired items'.

6. Various forms of realism have been argued for in recent years and perhaps the most influential has been that of critical realism (cf Bhaskar, 1979, 1989). A naive objectivist position argues that reality can be known by careful observation of patterns in social life. Bhaskar criticizes this position by making a distinction between epistemology and ontology. Our knowing of reality is always tentative, speculative and prone to error.

7. I have written about the self-referential element elsewhere (Scott, 1996a:147):

> Advocates of survey and correlational methods make a number of assumptions, the first of which is that a valid account of social interaction can be obtained, and the agenda for the investigation set, without reference being made to the way participants in the research understand and interpret their world. Research into race issues highlights this particular problem, since in much of the literature words such as 'race', 'immigrant', 'ethnic', 'black' and 'coloured' are employed as though they are neutral descriptive words...Race categories, it has been suggested, always incorporate a self-referential element. Those researchers who use pre-coded questionnaires necessarily make a number of assumptions about respondents which cannot be openly contested except by a refusal to take part in the exercise.

8. Macintyre (1988) suggests that these 'traditions of knowledge' are subject to dispute, reconfiguration and ultimately decay. However, for Macintyre, they are the source of all our knowledge.

9. These four positions – a-paradigmatic, di-paradigmatic, multi-paradigmatic and uni-paradigmatic – are ideal models and therefore contain within them a variety of other views.

10. For Hammersley (1992:8), ethnography can be equated with qualitative method: 'Throughout this book I use the term "ethnography" in a general sense, that is broadly equivalent to "qualitative research"'.

REFERENCES

Archer, M. (1982) Morphogenesis versus structuration. *British Journal of Sociology*, **33**(4), 455–483.

Ayer, A.J. (1936) *Knowledge, Truth and Logic*, London: Gollancz.

Bhaskar, R. (1979) *The Possibility of Naturalism*, Brighton: Harvester Press.

Bhaskar, R. (1989) *Reclaiming Reality*, London: Verso.

Bloom, B.S., Hastings, J.T. and Madaus, G.F. (1971) *Handbook on Formative and Summative Evaluation of Student Learning*, New York: McGraw-Hill.

Bryman (1988) *Quality and Quantity in Social Research*, London: Allen and Unwin.

Campbell, D.T. (1972) Reforms as experiments. In C.H. Weiss (ed.) *Evaluating Action Programmes: Reading in Social Action and Education*, Boston: Allyn and Bacon.

Cuckle, H.S. and Vunakis, H.V. (1984) The effectiveness of a postal smoking cessation kit. *Community Medicine*, **6**, 210–215.

Denzin, N. (1989) *Interpretive Interactionism, Vol. 16, Applied Social Research Methods*, London: Sage.

Denzin, N. and Lincoln, Y. (eds) (1995) *Handbook of Qualitative Research*, London: Sage.

Giddens, A. (1984) *The Constitution of Society*, Cambridge: Polity Press.

Glass, G.V. and Worthen, B.R. (1971) Evaluation and research: similarities and differences. *Curriculum Theory Network*, **Fall**, 149–165.

Guba, E. and Lincoln, Y. (1985) *Naturalistic Inquiry*, London: Sage.

Hammersley, M. (1992) *What's Wrong with Ethnography?* London: Routledge.

Herman, J.L., Morris, L.L. and Fitz-Gibbon, C.T. (1987) *Evaluator's Handbook*, London: Sage.

Kolakowski, L. (1975) *Husserl and the Search for Certitude*, New Haven: Yale University Press.

MacDonald, B. (1984) Evaluation and the control of education. In B. MacDonald and R. Walker (eds) *Innovation, Evaluation, Research and the Problem of Control (SAFARI)*, Norwich: CARE, University of East Anglia

Macintyre, A. (1988) *Whose Justice? Which Rationality?* London: Duckworth.

Naidoo, J. and Wills, J. (1994) *Health Promotion: Foundations for Practice*, London: Baillière Tindall.

Norris, N. (1992) *Understanding Educational Evaluation*, London: Kogan Page.

Patton, M.Q. (1986) *Utilization-focused Evaluation*, 2nd edn, Newbury Park: John Wiley

Scott, D. (1996a) Methods and data in educational settings. In D. Scott and R.Usher (eds) *Understanding Educational Research*, London: Routledge.

Scott, D. (1996b) Ethnography and education. In D. Scott and R. Usher (eds) *Understanding Educational Research*, London: Routledge.

Scriven, M. (1967) The methodology of evaluation. In American Educational Research Association, *Perspectives of Curriculum Evaluation*, Chicago: Rand McNally.

Simons, H. (1987) *Getting to Know Schools in a Democracy: The Politics and Process of Evaluation*, London: Falmer Press.

Smith, N.L. (1982) The context of evaluation practice in state departments of education. In Smith, N.L. and Caulley, D.N. (eds) *The Interaction of Evaluation and Policy: Case Reports from State Education Agencies*, Portland, Oregon: Northwest Regional Educational Laboratory (NREL).

Stake, R.E. (1967) The countenance of educational evaluation. *Teachers College Record*, **68**, 523–540

Stufflebeam, D.L., Foley, W.J., Gephart, W.J. *et al.* (1971) *Educational Evaluation and Decision Making*, Itasca, IL: Peacock

Tones, K., and Tilford, S. (1994) *Health Education: Effectiveness, Efficiency and Equity*, 2nd edition, London: Chapman and Hall.

Usher, R. (1993) *Reflexivity. Occasional Papers in Education and Interdisciplinary Studies*, No 3, Southampton: School of Education, University of Southampton.

Wolf, R.L. (1975) Trial by jury: a new evaluation method. *Phi Delta Kappa*, **57**(3), 185–218.

Effectiveness in health promotion: indicators and evidence of success

4

Keith Tones

Apart from the intrinsic importance of assessing programme effectiveness, economic constraints in both the health and education sectors have lead to managers and decision-makers demanding evidence that interventions actually work. Before discussing the nature of effectiveness, this chapter will examine the meaning of success for health promotion. It will define effectiveness, efficiency and efficacy and discuss the basis for selecting indicators for judging the extent to which programmes have met their objectives. It will raise questions about validity: about the basis on which we assess evidence of success. It will argue that a new standard of 'judicial review', based substantially on qualitative research techniques, should be preferred to the traditional research paradigms which adopt experimental design and the randomized controlled trial as a 'gold standard' of excellence.

Health promotion is a concept open to a number of sometimes conflicting interpretations. For instance, as we will see, the conceptualization developed by the World Health Organization (WHO) is quite different from the pragmatic operations which might be observed in UK primary care 'health promotion clinics' and, to a lesser extent, in the *Health of the Nation* policy (Department of Health, 1992). Logically it might be defined as any systematic attempt to promote health and prevent disease, but such a definition is too broad to be useful. A more limited definition will be provided later. At this point we will merely note that *health education* is more limited in its activities and aspirations than health promotion – of which it forms a significant part. Moreover, while definitions of health promotion give rise to philosophical debate, sometimes acrimonious, it is possible to offer a more technical definition of health education which is difficult to challenge. Further reference to health education in this chapter will be grounded in this definition.

> Health education is any intentional activity that is designed to achieve health- or illness- related learning, i.e. some relatively permanent change in an individual's capability or disposition. Thus, effective health education may produce changes in knowledge and understanding or ways of thinking; it may influence or clarify values; it may bring about some shift in belief or attitude; it may facilitate the acquisition of skills; it may even effect changes in behaviour or lifestyle (Tones, 1997: 786).

As we will see later, this definition incorporates a number of quite specific implications for selecting indicators of success.

PROGRAMME PLANNING AND THE RESEARCH PROCESS

Research should be an integral part of systematic health promotion planning and Figure 4.1 shows how this relates to the key features of the planning process. More particularly, research is concerned with:

1. determining the degree of priority which should be attached to a programme;
2. devising a preliminary 'educational diagnosis' of the target population;
3. appraising the degree of success or failure of the resulting programme.

As Figure 4.1 shows, effective health promotion programmes depend on a needs assessment involving a process of prioritization in which the programme in question competes for resources with other worthy causes. Assuming that the programme has been allocated a relatively high priority, its stated aims would, ideally, be translated into a list of highly specific objectives which are directly related to some target group or audience. Since a health promotion programme, as we will note below, is concerned with a synergistic combination of health education and 'healthy public policy', a health promotion intervention might well have both educational (or learning) objectives and policy objectives. Subsequently, interventions would be devised to achieve both categories of objective. Each of these would, of course, have identifiable content. In order to achieve programme goals, an appropriate methodology would be adopted: specific methods would be selected in order to achieve both the development and implementation of relevant policy and to facilitate learning in the target group. These methods will frequently be supported by the judicious selec-

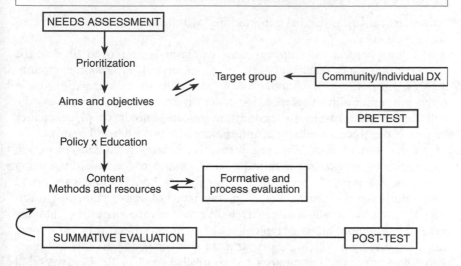

Figure 4.1   Health promotion: the place of research in planning the programme.

tion of audiovisual aids and other learning resources such as videos, models or teaching packs.

A more complete discussion of the programme planning process is available elsewhere (Tones and Tilford, 1994; Tones, 1993). For now we should merely note that the process of 'diagnosing' the characteristics of communities or individuals is not only an essential prerequisite for effective programme development but also serves to supply baseline data and at the same time act as a pretest which may be used in evaluating the intervention. The process of *summative evaluation* merely involves recording differences between *pre-* and *post-test* (and using appropriate techniques to allow claims to be made that any differences observed can be ascribed to the programme). *Formative evaluation*, on the other hand, monitors the programme and assesses its progress; it then uses the results of this assessment to make ongoing modifications and improvements. This developmental process can be applied to the programme as a whole or, more specifically, to the design and improvement of programme content.

Formative evaluation is central to *action research* – i.e. when the process of enquiry is concerned with the solution of social problems and data are used to make immediate changes which are, in turn, assessed for the effectiveness of their contribution to social change goals. Formative evaluation is also central to the notion of *mastery learning* (i.e. continually improving programme quality on the basis of formative assessment until some 90% of the target group achieve 90% of the levels of performance specified by the programme objectives). On a much smaller scale, formative evaluation (or developmental research) is commonly used for the development and refinement of mass media programmes within the broader context of *social marketing*.

The term *process evaluation* is now increasingly employed to describe the recording and documentation of a variety of programme circumstances: its purpose is illumination – especially to help explain why a given programme has succeeded or failed in achieving its objectives. We will argue later that health promotion research needs to place greater emphasis on process evaluation and, indeed, to move beyond it in pursuit of greater illumination. This argument also derives from the conviction that health promotion research must have a major concern with involving clients in the research process; accordingly, it should adopt rarely and with reluctance the neutral and arguably more objective stance of traditional, 'scientific' evaluation research. We will also be asserting that the need for illumination will typically cause us to reject this traditional research paradigm which adopts 'true experimental design' (or, in epidemiological parlance, the 'randomized controlled trial' or RCT) as its 'gold standard'.

EVALUATION AND THE MEANING OF SUCCESS: WHO VALUES WHAT?

Evaluation is essentially about determining the extent to which certain valued goals have been achieved and it is therefore meaningless to discuss whether or not a programme has been successful without first identifying these underlying values. It is not always apparent to research enthusiasts committed to the pursuit of scientific truth that there are usually a number of different stakeholders involved in the research process, and they may not subscribe to each other's values. Health services managers will often have different priorities from health workers. Politicians of all shapes and sizes will certainly have their own different priorities: their concern, ultimately, will be with re-election or having contracts renewed. Accordingly, their pressing interest in research results derives from a hunt for evidence to substantiate prejudice and/or support other political agendas, such as cutting resources from one programme in order to support another more favoured and politically beneficial course of action. We should also look out for the existence of different viewpoints within the ranks of health professionals and researchers themselves. The perspectives of medical practitioners may well be different from other health workers; 'traditional' epidemiologists may recoil from the methodologies of health sociologists who, themselves, may operate according to paradigms which differ from psychologists; advocates of health promotion may not see eye to eye with health educators. All of these may be out of tune with public interests and concerns. Those who believe that research is a neutral, detached and value-free scientific endeavour are likely to be severely disadvantaged in the fight for funding.

A full discussion of these different political and epistemological niceties is not possible here. We will, however, draw attention to one very important difference in stakeholder perspective by noting WHO's ideological position on health promotion and comparing this with the value focus of the medical model.

THE IDEOLOGY OF HEALTH PROMOTION

The key features of the medical model are well recognized: its focus is on disease, both treatment and prevention; its approach is reductionist and 'scientific'; its perspective has traditionally been 'top-down' with a requirement for people to *comply* with medical advice (Tones, in press). This is in sharp contrast to the World Health Organization's increasingly accepted ideology as enshrined in the Ottawa Charter (WHO, 1986). The values inherent in this ideology can be summarized thus.

- The pursuit of equity and the reduction of associated inequalities in health experience.
- A positive and holistic definition of health and a healthy society.
- An emphasis on *active participating communities* and *self-empowerment*. Empowerment is a desirable health goal in its own right; it is also the most effective means of dealing with the problems of premature and avoidable death and disease.
- A determination to achieve *demedicalization*: health is too important to leave to health professionals; the medical model tends to ignore the social and environmental determinants of health and traditional medical hegemony militates against empowerment.

In our search for evidence of success, we might therefore look for evidence of having achieved greater equity. For instance, to give the issue a UK flavour, we might ask what progress had been made in slaying William Beveridge's 'five giants of disease, idleness, ignorance, squalor and want'. We might also look for progress in people achieving self-reliance and in their capacity to control their own lives. We might search for signs of challenge to the 'culture of contentment' (Galbraith, 1992) by measuring levels of community indignation and concern about social pathogens which damage the quality of life and contribute to the inequitable distribution of disease and disability.

In short, health promotion programmes will have been successful insofar as they contribute to the explicit or implicit goals incorporated in the values statements listed above. Such broad goals are, of course, not only remarkably difficult to achieve but are also too general to be used as indicators of success and we will identify more specific proxy measures later. Further insights into the implications of health promotion ideology for the research and evaluation process are provided by Davies and Kelly (1993). At this juncture, however, and having commented on ideological matters, we will now consider implications for evaluation of the broad organizational structure of health promotion and its relationship with health education.

THE ANATOMY OF HEALTH PROMOTION

Ideology determines what is valued; anatomy describes the results of translating ideology into strategic practice. A more complete discussion is given in Tones (1997) but for now we will use a simple 'formula' which reminds us of the two essential elements of a health promotion programme, as outlined in Figure 4.1. In short:

Health promotion = health education × healthy public policy

Health education may have limited success without the support of 'healthy public policy' – an emblematic term accorded pride of place in the Ottawa Charter. In other words economic measures, legislation and environmental engineering are necessary to provide a 'supportive environment' in which 'the healthy choice is the easy choice'. For example, the adoption of a healthy diet will be considerably less difficult to achieve if healthy foods are available, readily accessible, clearly labelled and cheap. On the other hand, without health education, it is unlikely that the political barriers to the achievement of healthy public policy will be overcome. For instance, poverty is the major barrier to healthy eating. Governments are unlikely to seriously address the poverty of disadvantaged groups unless their political survival is threatened by popular outrage. Similarly, concerted parental pressure will dramatically increase school governors' conviction that their schools should adopt a fully fledged healthy eating policy to supplement nutrition education.

Health education thus has two major functions: first, it is concerned to empower *individual* health choices and second, it is concerned with *critical consciousness raising* – with creating a sense of public concern and indignation which leads to community action such that governments, organizations and others holding power are pressured into developing and implementing policies which promote health. Patton (1997) approvingly quotes Shah (1964: 58–59):

My Master taught me to spread the word that mankind will never be fulfilled until the man who has not been wronged is as indignant about a wrong as the man who actually has been wronged.

However, a codicil to the above quotation serves to remind us of the importance of our emotions being subject to critical appraisal of the facts before embarking on revolution:

> My Master taught me that nobody at all should become indignant about anything until he is sure that what he thinks is a wrong is in fact a wrong – and not a blessing in disguise.

It should be apparent, therefore, that the criteria for success in evaluating health promotion programmes will vary considerably according to whether stakeholders are basing their programme goals on a medical model of health promotion (according to WHO, a contradiction in terms) or are subscribing to the principles of the Ottawa Charter. Furthermore, we will also need to take account of the important synergy of policy and education in deciding what kind and degree of success we might expect from any given programme, i.e. its *effectiveness* and *efficiency*.

EVALUATION: EFFECTIVENESS, EFFICIENCY AND EFFICACY

Only a brief discussion of the complexities of evaluating health promotion programmes is possible in this chapter. For a more complete treatment, several useful texts are available – for instance, Green and Lewis (1986), Sarvela and McDermott (1993), Tones and Tilford (1994). Two broad criteria are typically used to determine the success of health promotion programmes: *effectiveness* and *efficiency*. Effectiveness simply refers to the extent to which a programme has achieved its goals whereas efficiency is a measure of *relative* effectiveness. In other words, efficiency describes the extent to which a given programme has achieved its goals by comparison with some alternative or competing intervention. For instance, if a course of drugs could lower population cholesterol levels more quickly and completely than dietary change, it would be a more efficient strategy. Again, it could well be the case that consistent and repeated price increases on cigarettes might be superior to education as a strategy for reducing tobacco consumption. Or, yet again, if health education delivered by the primary health care team could substantially lower the prevalence of smoking in teenage girls, it would be a more efficient procedure than building smoking education programmes into schools. By way of a final example, if we could show that a practice nurse using a *group discussion decision* method resulted in a higher rate of adoption and maintenance of breastfeeding than authoritative advice from a GP, then the group work would be judged to be the method of choice.

It is interesting to note that at the present time within the UK health services, there seems to be a shift in emphasis away from effectiveness and towards efficiency. This seems rather puzzling at first sight since in the terms discussed above, efficiency is a more rigorous measure of success. However, efficiency has often been used merely to refer to the relative effectiveness of a variety of different *inputs* to the health care system, arguably at the expense of ignoring whether these inputs actually resulted in effective *outcomes*. In the field of health promotion and education in general, efficiency should, according to many programme planners, always be linked to specified outcomes in the form of *aims* (general statements of intent) and *objectives* (much more specific specifications of outcome). Indeed, as we will see, objectives which state specific *learning* outcomes, by definition, incorporate a measure of efficiency in that they are expected to indicate both the conditions under which the learning is to be demonstrated and the *standard* to be achieved (Mager, 1962).

Although there is no universal agreement, the term 'efficacy' is increasingly added to the concepts of effectiveness and efficiency. It is used here to refer to the efficient and effective achievement of goals *under ideal conditions*. Since efficacy has important implications for judgements about the validity of traditional research designs, we will revisit this concept later in the chapter.

OBJECTIVES, EFFICIENCY AND STANDARDS OF SUCCESS

Aims, then, are general statements of intent. The over-riding aim of health promotion might be described as *health gain*, which embodies the tripartite goal of:

- adding years to life – reducing avoidable death;
- adding health to life – reducing disease and disability;
- adding life to years – enhancing the quality of life.

Although these broad aims may serve an inspirational purpose, they must be translated into much more specific goals before a programme can be constructed with precision and accuracy and before it can be convincingly evaluated. Accordingly, systematically designed programmes will translate their aims into objectives. These objectives will be more specific than the aims from which they have been developed. Indeed, it is not uncommon now to use the acronym SMART as a guide for the production of objectives. Objectives should therefore be:

S　Specific
M　Measurable
A　Achievable
R　Realistic
T　Timescale (should be stated).

In health promotion, we can distinguish operational or policy objectives from educational objectives. The former would describe the specific goals to be attained in the development and implementation of policy while the latter would be concerned with the specific outcomes which should result if a health *education* programme is successful.

The following examples from the Health Promotion Authority Wales (1992) illustrate both kinds of objective.

Policy objectives

- Increase to over 95% those who have received personal, health and social education (including sex education) at school as part of the planned curriculum.
- Increase to over 50% those who receive the positive support of another person when attempting to give up smoking, lose weight, take more exercise or reduce alcohol.
- Increase to over 95% those hospitals which have fully implemented policies: (1) restricting smoking in all public areas, (2) promoting healthy catering.
- Reduce to less than 1% the number of houses without basic amenities.

Educational objectives

- Increase to at least 90% those who understand the essential element of the European Code for cancer prevention.
- Increase to over 95% those who consider that not smoking should be the normal way of living.
- Decrease to less than 5% those who show prejudice against people with AIDS or HIV.
- Increase to over 96% those who would like to lose weight, reduce alcohol consumption, take more exercise, stop smoking.

Again, objectives themselves can vary in degree of specificity. However our discussion here will centre on the most precise and rigorous variety – the *behavioural* learning objective. The subject is relevant to the purpose of this chapter in that it illustrates a device which can enhance the efficiency of programme planning and provide a sound basis for reliable and valid evaluation. It also illustrates the value dimension underpinning what at first sight seems to be a merely technical matter.

We can usefully envisage aims and objectives being distributed on a kind of spectrum of specificity. For instance, the general (epidemiological) aim of reducing the prevalence of lung cancer in women might be translated into a rather more specific aim – to reduce the onset of smoking in teenage girls. This in turn might be translated into an objective, such as 'to help young women resist pressure from friends to smoke an unwanted cigarette'. A behavioural objective, on the other hand, is more specific still and must always focus on the learner's performance rather than the teacher's. Not only must it translate any kind of learning into observable behaviour (e.g. 'will *list* the harmful effects of smoking'), it must also state the *conditions* leading to this demonstration of learning and the *standard* to be achieved. An example of a social interaction skills learning objective is provided below.

Young people aged 16 who havealready demonstrated their understanding of the principles of assertiveness	The Learners
having participated in role play exercise 1B in a youth club setting	Conditions
will assertively refuse an offer of a cigarette using appropriate eye contact, facial expression, posture and voice modulation.	Behaviours
Learners will score at least 4 on a five-point peer-rating scale.	Standards of sucess

At first sight, it might appear that a behavioural objective may only be appropriate for overt behaviours, such as routine actions like smoking a cigarette or for psychomotor or social interaction skills. However, advocates of learning objectives insist that it is possible to write objectives for all cognitive and affective outcomes – in fact, for all the variables which we will later describe as 'intermediate' and 'indirect' indicators of success.

Writing behavioural objectives can have a very salutary effect in sharpening thinking processes. However, apart from the advantages of specificity, they offer two further benefits to evaluators. These derive from their incorporating the conditions under which a given learned outcome is to be demonstrated and the standards which have to be met if the learning is to be judged successful. The former requirement reminds us that a given learning outcome will only be achieved if the conditions necessary for any learning situation have been fulfilled. In the example provided above, the acquisition of social interaction skill requires repeated practice together with feedback; the method of choice might be guided practice, with or without video analysis and/or role play. The importance of ensuring minimum conditions for success will be mentioned later in our discussion of *efficacy*. The matter of standards is also relevant to this concept and perhaps needs some further comment here.

In brief, any programme planner should decide on how well the programme should perform if it is to be considered successful. Green and Lewis (1986) identified four levels of success: *historical, normative, theoretical* and *absolute*. Historical standards are applied when the planner merely judges relative success by comparing results with the level of success achieved in previous ventures of a similar kind. Normative standards are somewhat similar in that the level of performance is judged by comparing it with how well similar programmes operated by other health promoters under comparable circumstances performed. Theoretical standards are derived from expectations based on theory. For instance, the Health Action Model (Tones, 1987; Tones and Tilford, 1994) might show, *inter alia*, that a number of beliefs about susceptibility and seriousness need to be complemented by beliefs about self-efficacy. Furthermore, the individual in question might also need to accept that she would probably be able to cope with loss of gratification and the anticipated 'withdrawal symptoms' associated with giving up smoking before she would seriously consider quitting. In addition, a relatively high level of self-esteem would be helpful and various supportive skills and a favourable environment would be necessary before her intention to give up smoking could be translated into practice. Expectations of success would be proportional to the extent that some or all of these theoretically prescribed conditions had been fulfilled.

Green and Lewis contrast the three categories of standard mentioned above with a fourth standard of success. This demands nothing less than perfection, i.e. 100% success. While not demanding quite such high standards, politicians and sponsors do tend to make decidedly unrealistic demands on health promoters. A preliminary political task, therefore, is to try to generate an appreciation of the complexities of most interventions and seek to reduce the more extreme ambitions of funding bodies.

OBJECTIVES AND PROFESSIONAL VALUES

We noted earlier the different values and perspectives which may exist among different stakeholders in the research process, including professionals. The enthusiasm for behavioural objectives is a case in point. Popham (1978) discussed the rise and fall of a 'behavioural objectives movement' on certain US university campuses in the 1960s. He described an adversarial bumper sticker which read '*Help stamp out non-behavioural objectives!*'. Such energetic enthusiasm by the pro-objectives lobby was inevitably countered by an extreme aversion to objectives on the part of advocates of other educational approaches. It is not possible here to describe the complexities of the debate but opponents of the objectives movement tend to argue that it is not possible to translate their own sophisticated activities into anything so crude as observable behaviours, and a focus on behavioural objectives can blind the evaluator to other and possibly more important results of a given programme. The first observation doubtless relates to Patton's (1997) observation that probably half the population is guilty of 'fuzzy conceptualizing'. It *is* possible, though often exceedingly difficult, to write behavioural objectives for any taught activity; if it is not, then it will be impossible to evaluate it with any degree of certainty. As Mager (1962) noted: 'If you do not know where you are going, you will probably never get there!'.

It is even possible and desirable to negotiate objectives with client groups in the context of community development (at least in its purest form) since, by definition, the participatory process cannot start with a statement of specific objectives but must be based on the community's identification of its own 'felt needs'. The second observation is undoubtedly more significant: in conditions of uncertainty we would certainly not use specific objectives but would seek to develop understandings of the ways in which target groups view their world. However, this latter kind of research is not evaluation research. On the other hand, the assessment of unanticipated programme effects in evaluation research *is* a necessary part of the research endeavour and requires the use of appropriately designed formative and process evaluation – which may result in objectives being rewritten, reinvented or even completely discarded.

ON COST EFFECTIVENESS

One of the most important criteria for appraising the efficiency of programme interventions involves calculating the relative financial costs of competing interventions (*cost-effectiveness analysis*). *Cost-benefit analysis*, on the other hand, not only states the costs in monetary terms but also seeks to place a price tag on the benefits accruing from the programme. A calculation of the cost per given benefit is then possible (typically expressed as a cost-benefit ratio). Now, on the one hand, there is quite firm evidence that health promotion can achieve results which demonstrate not only cost effectiveness but also commendable cost-benefit ratios. On the other hand, cost effectiveness can be a double-edged weapon. We will provide some brief elaboration of these assertions but we might note that cost is by no means always used as a criterion for action. Mooney (1977) demonstrated the truth of this observation quite convincingly when he showed that the cost per life saved for a variety of preventive measures ranged from £50 per life saved for stillbirth screening to £20 million per life saved for alterations to high-rise flats after the Ronan Point disaster.

As long ago as 1974, Green showed how a specific health education programme resulted in a saving of $7.81 per dollar invested in a hypertension screening and education programme; he also demonstrated that using group discussion techniques to educate asthmatic patients about the best means of controlling their condition notched up a cost-benefit ratio of 1:5. More recently, a British study of the effectiveness of family planning service (Laing, 1982) identified conservative benefit-to-cost ratios of 1.3:1 for preventing 'typical unplanned pregnancies'; a ratio of 4.5:1 for preventing pregnancies among mothers of three or more children; a 5.3:1 ratio for unplanned, premarital conceptions. As the author put it: '...for every £100 spent on family planning services, the public sector can expect a benefit of £130, £450 and £530 respectively'.

In relation to smoking education programmes, Townsend (1986) argued that if a hypothetical mass media programme were to result in 1000 people giving up smoking permanently, 10,000 giving up temporarily, 2000 cutting down and 15,000 seriously considering giving up, then 2991 life years would be saved at a cost of £84 per life. This is admittedly a hypothetical example but Phillips and Prowle (1993) offered a more tangible analysis of benefits by calculating the costs and benefits of the 'Heartbeat Wales' programme. They were unable, for reasons to be explored later, to precisely ascribe cause and effect. However, on a pessimistic, 'worst case' assumption that the programme had only a 10% impact rate on the *actual* decline in smoking in Wales over a four-year period (1985–1989), they estimated that the, 'net cost per working life year saved ... worked out at approximately £64'. Warner (1994) also makes the following observation (in a US context):

> In the absence of the anti-smoking campaign, adult per capita cigarette consumption in 1987 would have been an estimated 78–89% higher than the level actually experienced. .... As a result, ... an estimated 789,200 Americans avoided or postponed smoking-related deaths and gained an average of 21 additional years of life expectancy each.

Finally, recent studies in UK have demonstrated the efficiency of GPs providing advice to stop smoking in accordance with quite stringent economic criteria. For a budget of £1 million a relatively straightforward and simple intervention has been calculated to 'notch up' some 59,888 quality-adjusted life years (QALYs) compared with, for example, a much lower figure for breast screening (302 QALYs). Again, it is generally considered that hip replacement is a highly efficient and appropriate surgical procedure yet it costs £750 per QALY compared with £167 for GP-provided, smoking-related advice (Godfrey *et al.*, 1989).

Despite this cheering evidence of effectiveness, economic indicators of success should be treated with caution. Even allowing for 'discounting' – the process whereby future costs are considered less important than current costs – it seems likely that really effective health promotion will postpone death and contribute to an increasingly large elderly population. In the last analysis, this will increase the substantial medical costs involved in treating very old people as well as increasing the pensions and benefits bill. Perhaps the most useful approach to this dilemma is to follow the recommendations made by Cohen (1981). Prevention (and health promotion) should be treated as a 'merit good', i.e. something which satisfies a 'merit want'. According to Musgrave (cited by Cohen, 1981), merit wants are, '... so meritorious that their satisfaction is provided for through the public budget over and above what is provided for through the market and paid for by private buyers'. Clearly, such a view has especial significance at this time in the development of thinking about health services and the market place. At all events, health promotion can demonstrate its capacity to satisfy quite stringent measures of efficiency. However, we need to examine more critically which indicators of its effectiveness and efficiency are most appropriate for those seeking to evaluate success.

INDICATORS OF SUCCESS

We have thus far discussed the meaning of success and the three broad criteria for assessing how well programmes have achieved their goals, i.e. effectiveness, efficiency and efficacy. We also pointed out that the broad value-laden goals of health promotion, or even a preventive medical model, must be translated into more specific indicators of success. We will now consider the nature of such indicators and the basis for selecting them. We will first challenge what for many people is epidemiological orthodoxy by questioning the value of certain kinds of outcome measure.

Limitations of outcome measures

Some of the practical and philosophical perspectives of different stakeholders, which were mentioned earlier, may be seen in decision-making about the kinds of indicator which might be used as measures of the success, or otherwise, of health promotion programmes. Other influences on the appropriate choice of indicator are purely practical. For one or more reasons, outcome measures are frequently inappropriate and the effectiveness and efficiency of health promotion programmes must be assessed by two categories of proxy indicators which will be described here as indirect and intermediate indicators.

Our first contention is that epidemiological indicators should *never* be used in evaluating health promotion. In the first place, it is frequently impracticable to measure the success of even a preventive medical intervention in terms of reductions in mortality or morbidity since the impact of the programme might not be apparent for several years. More fundamentally, the only medical justification for seeking to influence people's behaviours and lifestyles is if there is a demonstrable relationship between those behaviours and that lifestyle and the negative health outcomes.

Unless these links are robust, it is not only inefficient to mount a programme, it is unethical. If the association is not proven or is uncertain, *epidemiological* research needs to be done in order to demonstrate that behaviour change is likely to reduce risk. Accordingly, the 'hardest' outcome measure of programme effectiveness will be the adoption of preventive behaviours and/or a change in those aspects of lifestyle which have been shown to prevent disease at primary, secondary or tertiary levels. Even then, behavioural outcomes will frequently be inappropriate for assessing programme success.

The proximal–distal chain and intermediate indicators

It is useful to consider the relationship between health promotion inputs and outputs in terms of a succession of often complex and interacting series of temporal events. Figure 4.2 provides some explanation for this requirement by considering how a number of beliefs about cancer might influence a hypothetical individual's decision to seek early medical advice with a skin lesion.

As Tones and Tilford (1994:94) observe:

Before seeking medical assistance, the individual in question must first recognize that (s)he has a skin lesion. She must then believe it might be skin cancer, i.e. she must form a level of subjective probability which justifies a visit to her doctor ... The individual's belief about the likelihood of the sore on her hand being skin cancer will be influenced by her pre-existing belief about her susceptibility to that

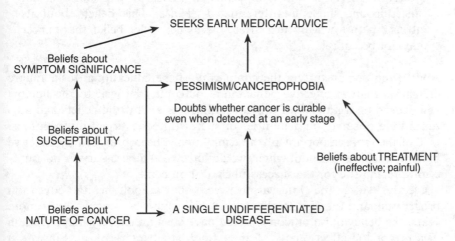

Figure 4.2 Contributions of beliefs to decision to seek medical advice.

disease (which, in turn, will depend on her understanding and beliefs about the risk factors). Her intention to visit her doctor will also be influenced by her belief about the seriousness of the disease. Now, according to the Health Belief Model (Becker, 1984), the product of susceptibility and seriousness is a particular level of perceived threat. However, ... too high a level of fear generated by that perception of threat may give rise to defensive avoidance rather than 'rational' action. It is for that reason that it may be better if the individual ... should have only a moderate level of conviction about the likelihood of her particular lesion being cancer: a very high level of certainty may create too high a level of arousal and give rise to delay in service utilization....

[Figure 2] shows cancerophobia (which derives from the general belief system which we label 'pessimism') as a significant barrier to action. ... this barrier derives from a number of subordinate beliefs, one of which is the belief that treatment for cancer is (i) generally ineffective and (ii) painful or distressing...

Again, we need to probe further before structuring our education programme. We need to ask about the origin of these 'higher order' beliefs. If we do so, we realise that we must consider beliefs about the nature of cancer and its causes. For instance, it has been well documented that people may have a variety of 'theories' about the cause of cancer. A retribution theory considers that cancer has been visited on the individual as a punishment for past moral transgressions. The 'seed and trigger theory' posits that we all have cancer within us in a dormant form, like a kind of seed, which is merely waiting for some event (almost any event – a knock, death in the family, work stress) to trigger it. ... It (also) appears that many people consider that cancer is one single undifferentiated disease. This belief about its intrinsic nature will in turn affect the higher order belief that cancer may not be curable.

Apart from demonstrating the complexity of the educational task, Figure 4.2 shows that an effective behavioural outcome (the visit to the doctor) will depend on a number of previous influences and, if the beliefs and attitudes were positive, on a number of successful educational interventions. One of the more important of these might have been provided by effective biology teaching in school which would have been a necessary, if not sufficient, prerequisite for the successful clinical outcome.

Clearly, since the interval between the school health education programme and the visit to the doctor might have been some 40 or more years, the behavioural outcome would have been an entirely inappropriate measure of the effectiveness of the school-based intervention. Since it is important to evaluate school programmes, different indicators would have to be used. In fact, evaluating pupils' knowledge and beliefs about cancer would use outcome indicators of the effectiveness of the biology programme but would be an intermediate indicator of the effectiveness of a longer term skin cancer programme. It is useful, therefore, to think of a kind of 'proximal–distal' chain of health promotion interventions and associated *intermediate indicators* of success.

Furthermore, it is important to emphasise the fact that successful health promotion rarely involves the administration of a 'one-off' input. Not only does it involve a number of different kinds of educational intervention at different times but, as we noted earlier, it also involves the provision of policy measures designed to create a supportive environment which will maximize the chance of health education success. For instance, education about non-smoking will be more effective in a context in which advertising has been banned and smoking does not happen in public places. Utilization of cervical cytology screening or mammography services requires an efficient call and recall system and a generally user-friendly environment.

We might also note, in passing, that certain variables might be viewed as intermediate indicators of success in a programme whose objectives are to achieve preventive outcomes while at the same time being considered as outcome indicators by those seeking to achieve the major Ottawa goal of empowerment. For instance, the acquisition of assertiveness skills could be seen as a worthwhile empowerment and mental health goal in its own right but be considered a *prerequisite* for adopting preventive actions such as refusing drugs or unwanted sex.

Indirect indicators

Before leaving the concept of the proximal–distal chain, we should also note the need for a separate category of indicator, here referred to as *indirect indicators*. In short, we frequently need to evaluate interventions which make a relatively distal but essential contribution to outcomes. For instance, a mass media message must be pretested and modified before being broadcast (as indicated in Figure 4.1). A training course designed to equip teachers with the knowledge, skills and motivation to use a cancer education package with young people in school must be evaluated if it is to be improved and adopted.

Figure 4.3 provides an overview of the proximal–distal chain, together with its associated indicators in the context of an analysis of key programme components designed to increase the likelihood of women's use of cytology services. The epidemiological indicator – reduced incidence of cervical cancer – is included in the diagram but, as mentioned previously, should not be considered an indicator *of health promotion* success.

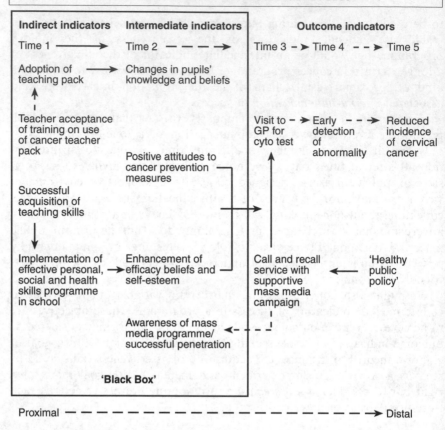

Figure 4.3 Indicators of success: the proximal–distal chain (MacDonald, Veen and Tones, 1996; reproduced with permission).

Which indicator?

Given the complexities of health promotion interventions and their distribution over an often quite lengthy period of time, a wide variety of different indicators will be used. Table 4.1 provides a list of types of indicator derived from the Health Action Model.

On what basis should these various indicators be selected? The answer is, in principle at least, very simple. We already have a substantial theoretical understanding of both the psychosocial and environmental factors which determine people's decisions to adopt and maintain healthy (or unhealthy) choices – see, for instance, the Health Action Model mentioned above (Tones, 1997; Tones and Tilford, 1994) – and also of the theoretical basis for choosing educational and pedagogical methods.

Table 4.1 Health action model and indicators of success

- Knowledge and understanding
- Effective educational provision
- Beliefs: causal attributions; nature of disease; theories of illness
- Beliefs about susceptibility: seriousness; benefits and costs
- Beliefs about social norms: anticipated reactions of significant others
- Beliefs about self: self-concept; body image; self efficacy; cognitive, decisional and contingency control; existential control
- Source credibility and associated attributes
- Affective: values and attitudes
- Emotional states: positive/negative affect/gratification (and beliefs about these); guilt, embarrassment, dissonance, anxiety, fear
- 'Personality': sensation seeking; locus of control; self-esteem
- Normative factors: social norms; cultural beliefs and values; stigma of diseases; social structure/community network
- Skills: psychomotor; self-regulatory; social interaction
- Behavioural intentions: level of probability of readiness to act; stage of change
- Behavioural outcomes: choices; sustained behaviour changes and routines; lifestyle; relapse
- Environment: macro, meso and micro; state of policy development and implementation
- Environment: levels of social support

A final word on the utility of thinking in terms of a proximal–distal chain of effects in relation to our earlier observations about standard setting is appropriate. If a successful outcome depends on the satisfactory negotiation of a succession of psychosocial and environmental tasks, then the greater the number of such links in this proximal–distal chain, the greater the effort which will be needed to attain the final goal and the less likely it is that success will be achieved. This has been described in social marketing parlance as a hierarchy of communication effects. Table 4.2 provides a hypothetical example of this phenomenon in relation to a community-wide marketing campaign. It shows that ultimate success is only 1.04% product sales. Since health promotion often seeks to sell rather unpalatable products, it is important not to set our sights too high.

EVALUATION OF EFFECTIVENESS AND EFFICIENCY: SELECTING APPROPRIATE RESEARCH METHODOLOGY

An extensive discussion of research design is inappropriate here. However, following earlier observations about the requirements of the WHO's approach to health promotion and the potential disagreements and even conflict between different stakeholders, it is important to make a number of assertions which centre on (i) the inappropriateness of traditional

Table 4.2   The hierarchy of communication effects

Attracts and sustains attention
Message recognized and main points recalled   =   65%
Message fully understood

Customers believe message and consider it
personally relevant
Customers do not perceive any major barriers   =   20%
involved in using product
Customers have positive attitude to buying product

Environment is conducive to sales and customer has   =   40%
necessary skills to use it

Customers take action and buy product   =   40%
(cf. make healthy choice)

Customers continue to buy product   =   50%
(cf. healthy choice routinized)

In short, the proportion sustaining the behaviour change   =
            (65% × 20% × 40% × 40% × 50%) × 100 =   **1.04%**

research designs – particularly the randomized controlled trial (RCT) – and (ii) the need for a new 'gold standard' which is grounded in illuminative methodology and utilizes triangulation to provide a new kind of 'judicial' evidence.

The limitations of the RCT

We are at present witnessing a demand for *evidence-based medicine* within a general climate of cost cutting and a concern to demonstrate '*health gain*'. We should, however, note that within health services in general, it is quite unusual to base practice on hard evidence (Brook and Lohr, 1985). Indeed, if we accept the premises on which Warner's (1994) '*health gain rhomboid*' are based, only 20% of all health care interventions have been validated using the 'gold standard' of the randomized controlled trial (RCT). According to Warner, an equal proportion have been shown to be of no value, while the remainder have 'uncertain effects'.

The RCT (or its educational equivalent, the true experimental design) is still considered to provide the 'gold standard' for evaluation studies. The behavioural science/educational equivalent is the 'true experimental design'. Both of these are problematical and typically inappropriate for evaluating health promotion programmes and, according to some (Charlton, 1991), are not always even appropriate for assessing clinical interventions. The main critique centres on the following points.

- They are difficult to achieve in practice.
- Random allocation is difficult and artificial.
- There are often ethical issues in withholding health promotion from individuals and communities.
- Contamination is almost inevitable when trying to compare experimental areas with control or comparison areas in large-scale interventions. For instance, Nutbeam *et al.* (1990), commenting on the design of a Welsh heart disease prevention programme, demonstrated that within a matter of weeks, the control region was heavily engaged in its own heart health initiatives.
- Health promotion (as we noted above) usually involves a complex multifactorial intervention; it is dramatically different from the provision of medication, for which the RCT might well be suitable.
- It is ideologically unsound for health promotion; we cannot treat people as objects. Health promotion *research*, like health promotion generally, requires individual and community *participation* and associated *action research*. As Raeburn (1987: 2, cited by Vanderplaat, 1995) says: 'Community people decide what their own needs are, set their own goals, and take action themselves ... these projects are owned, controlled and determined by the people whom they are intended to benefit ... at the heart of the system is a fundamental principle, that of people deciding what they want for themselves'.
- Traditional research designs provide minimal illumination; we might learn that a given intervention has been successful or has failed but we would normally not know why. Admittedly, the recognition of this problem is leading to a stipulation that programmes should have at least some *process evaluation* included. A lack of illuminative evidence can create a particular dilemma for managers responsible for commissioning services and programmes: the RCT typically provides hard evidence for decision-making about whether to commit resources to particular 'proven' programmes but does not explain just what constitutes effectiveness nor provides even minimal guidelines on how to implement such programmes.

A TALE OF THREE ERRORS: ILLUMINATION AND THE JUDICIAL PRINCIPLE

The notion of type I and type II error is very familiar to researchers working in the logical positivist paradigm. Type I error results when unjustifiable claims are made for the success of a programme, typically because inadequate controls have been established to allow programme planners to claim that changes in the target group are due to programme effects rather than external 'contaminating' factors. Type II errors occur when, for example, the measuring instruments used (e.g. inappropriate or inadequately validated self-esteem scales) are insufficiently sensitive to detect the existence of real changes which are in fact due to the health promotion intervention. Type III error refers to a tendency to deny the effectiveness of a health promotion programme when that programme was inadequately designed and therefore doomed to fail. A similar phenomenon has been observed in the world of computing and has been encapsulated in the acronym *GIGO* – *'garbage in, garbage out'*.

For instance, a community-wide smoking prevention programme might require a synergistic approach involving both policy change and education before it might be expected to show results. A successful face-to-face encounter between health professional and client would require the use of proven counselling techniques plus the involvement of support groups with family members before significant dietary changes might occur in the target group of middle-aged, overweight men. To judge the effectiveness of health promotion on the basis of a brief and unskilled encounter in which a doctor advises the patient to lose weight is, I suspect, not uncommon. However, this does a major disservice to health promotion and commits the unpardonable type III error.

Efficacy and type III error

Unfortunately, attempts to deal with type III error may result in a paradox: to develop and refine a programme until it nears perfection and then evaluate it can lead to real difficulties due to the fact that it may well be far too difficult and expensive in real life to provide the conditions necessary to replicate ideal-type programmes. Accordingly, the results of a demonstration project which mobilizes the resources needed to provide effective health promotion, and thus avoid type III error, will lack *external validity* in that it will not be possible to generalize from the experience and therefore ordinary practitioners in normal circumstances will not be able to reproduce the programme, even though it has been demonstrably effective in an experimental situation.

There are two important implications for evaluating health promotion practice. First (as we noted earlier), assessing a given health promotion programme when this has not been developed and implemented in accordance with best practice (i.e. under ideal conditions) can lead to type III error. On the other hand, to develop and refine a programme until it nears perfection and then evaluate it can also lead to difficulties. Since ideal circumstances can rarely if ever be achieved outside the laboratory, insistence on efficacy measures can militate against external validity, i.e. it would not be possible to generalize from the experience. Nonetheless, since a wide variety of health promotion programmes (dare one say when they have been operated by the untrained and uninitiated) often fall so far short of perfection that failure can be almost guaranteed, a compromise position must be identified. The implication is doubtless obvious:

1. determine the kinds of result which might be expected from different levels and sophistication of input;
2. decide on a threshold below which it is worthless running a programme;
3. be sure to build quality standards into programme objectives.

As we mentioned earlier, *force majeure* in the form of a political imperative may result in the launch of an ill-considered and ill-resourced campaign. The solution to this little difficulty is quite simple – in theory. Different objectives should be devised which centre on the achievement of political rather than health promotion goals.

THE NEED FOR ILLUMINATION AND THE QUESTION OF VALIDITY

Before arguing the case for illuminative evaluation, it is essential to acknowledge the need to pursue validity vigorously. To opt for qualitative techniques does not mean abandoning validity – quite the reverse. We might also acknowledge that it is *possible* to use complex variations on the RCT or, more accurately, on true experimental designs in order to gain some degree of illumination. For instance, complex multivariate analysis might tease out the relative contributions of the multitude of factors which are necessary, if not sufficient, to achieve programme success and which operate synergistically in the ways discussed above. However, such an approach would be ponderous and require innumerable repetitious studies before some degree of illumination is provided. Moreover, it would be virtually impossible using such a strategy – which tends to use quantitative methods – to gain real insights into the complex and often contradictory world of people's beliefs and feelings (on which health decisions are based). In short, the alternative paradigm is preferred.

Triangulation and the use of evidence

As mentioned above, the validity of illuminative research must be rigorously addressed. In fact, given its current low status in the medical research hegemony, the question of validity must be paramount. Accordingly, I would argue that we should assemble evidence of success using a kind of 'judicial principle', by which I mean providing evidence which would lead to a jury committing themselves to take action even though 100% proof is not available. The well-recognized technique for providing such evidence is that of *triangulation*. Triangulation involves accumulating evidence from a variety of sources; if the resulting data all point in the same direction, it is reasonable to assume that a programme has been successful and the insights gained from the documentation of process (which is central to the whole operation) can be used to repeat and improve on the interventions in question.

The main elements of triangulation have been fully explored by Denzin (1978). Data triangulation includes:

- investigator triangulation;
- theory triangulation;
- methodological triangulation.

Janesick (1994) adds an additional dimension: 'interdisciplinary triangulation'. Why should we not, for example, use data from other disciplines, such as art or literature, to support our behavioural and social science conclusions? The notion of triangulation is not really that radical. Let us consider the generally accepted criteria for inferring cause in medicine:

- a strong association;
- a dose–response relationship;
- association should be:
    consistent
    specific
    temporally correct
    biologically plausible.

A similar checklist can operate for health promotion, with one or two modifications. For instance, the dose–response relationship would relate to the better results achieved by appropriate synergistic interventions and the notion of biological plausibility would be replaced by *theoretical plausibility* in relation to social, psychological and pedagogical practice.

CONCLUSION

This chapter has inevitably been somewhat simplistic and has avoided one issue frequently debated by research theorists, some of whom would argue on epistemological grounds that logical positivism *per se* (and therefore the whole splendid edifice of the hypothetico-deductive system) has no place in health promotion. There are those who would fundamentally challenge the medical model. The view presented here, however, involves compromise. In Voltaire's words, the author is, '...*un homme pour qui le monde existe*!'. He believes that it is certainly very worthwhile to prevent disease. Moreover, an underlying assumption in this chapter is that the Ottawa Charter principles are compatible with the prevention of disease, provided only that medicine embraces the principle of empowerment and abandons its traditional top-down approach. The implications for researching health promotion have hopefully been made clear. We must above all emphasize illumination and assemble evidence of success using whatever methods are available: methodological pluralism is not only acceptable but essential. We need to pursue validity rigorously and be inventive in triangulating evidence for success. There are, of course, barriers to be overcome: for instance, the conservatism of some of the professions associated with delivering and researching health promotion; the still powerful medical hegemony and its authoritarian emphasis on a top-down approach; and politicians.

Of these, perhaps the greatest barrier is the political imperative. As Galbraith (1992) noted in his masterly discussion of the 'culture of contentment': 'A final word on politics. As in economics, nothing is certain save the certainty that there will be firm prediction by those who do not know!'.

REFERENCES

Becker, M.H. (ed.) (1984) *The Health Belief Model and Personal Health Behaviour*, New York: Charles B. Slack.

Brook, R. and Lohr, K. (1985) Efficiency, effectiveness, variations and quality. *Medical Care*, **23**, 710–722.

Charlton, B.G. (1991) Medical practice and the double-blind, randomized controlled trial. *British Journal of General Practice*, **September**, 355–356.

Cohen, D. (1981) *Prevention as a Merit Good*, Aberdeen: Health Economics Research Unit, University of Aberdeen.

Davies, J.K. and Kelly, M.P. (1993) *Healthy Cities: Research and Practice*, London: Routledge.

Denzin, N.K. (1978) *The Research Act: a Theoretical Introduction to Sociological Methods*, 2nd edn, New York: McGraw-Hill.

Department of Health (1992) *Health of the Nation*, London: HMSO.

Galbraith, J.K. (1992) *The Culture of Contentment*, Harmondsworth: Penguin.

Godfrey, C., Hardman, G. and Maynard, A. (1989) *Priorities for Health Promotion: An Economic Approach*, Discussion Paper 59, York: Centre for Health Economics, University of York.

Green, L.W. (1974) Toward cost-benefit evaluation of health education: some concepts, methods and examples. *Health Education Monographs*, **2**, 34–64.

Green, L.W. and Lewis, F.M. (1986) *Assessment and Evaluation in Health Education and Health Promotion*, Palo Alto, CA: Mayfield.

Health Promotion Authority Wales (1992) *Health Promotion: Challenges for the 1990s*, Cardiff: HPAW.

Janesick, V.J. (1994) The dance of qualitative research design: metaphor, methodolatry and meaning. In N.K. Denzin and Y.S. Lincoln (eds) *Handbook of Qualitative Research*, London: Sage.

Laing, W.A. (1982) *Family Planning: the Benefits and Costs*, No. 607, London: Policy Studies Institute.

Macdonald, G., Veen, C. and Tones, K. (1996) Evidence for success in health promotion: suggestions for improvement. *Health Education Research*, **11**(3): 367–376.

Mager, R.F. (1962) *Preparing Instructional Objectives*, Belmont, CA: Fearon.

Mooney, G.H. (1977) *The Valuation of Human Life*, London: Macmillan.

Nutbeam, D., Smith, C., Murphy, S. and Catford, J. (1990) Maintaining evaluation designs in long term community based health promotion programmes: Heartbeat Wales Study. *Journal of Epidemiology and Community Health*, **47**, 127–133.

Patton, M.W. (1997) *Utilization-Focused Evaluation*, Thousand Oaks: Sage.

Phillips, C.J. and Prowle, M.J. (1993) Economics of a reduction in smoking: case study from Heartbeat Wales. *Journal of Epidemiology and Community Health*, **47**, 215–223.

Popham, W.J. (1978) Must all objectives be behavioural? In D. Hamilton and M. Parlett (eds) *Beyond the Numbers Game*, London: Macmillan.

Raeburn, J. (1987) People projects: planning and evaluation in a new era. *Health Promotion*, **winter**, 2–13.

Sarvela, P.D. and McDermott, R.J. (1993) *Health Education Evaluation and Measurement: a Practitioner's Perspective*, Madison, WI: Brown and Benchmark.

Shah, I. (1964) *The Sufis*, New York: Doubleday.

Tones, B.K. (1987) Devising strategies for preventing drug misuse: the role of the health action model. *Health Education Research*, **2**, 305–318.

Tones, B.K. (1993) Changing theory and practice: trends in methods, strategies and settings in health education. *Health Education Journal*, **52**(3), 126–139.

Tones, B.K. (1997) Health education, behaviour change and the public health. In R. Dettels and J. McEwen (eds) *Oxford Textbook of Public Health*, Oxford: OUP.

Tones, B.K. (in press) Health promotion: empowering choice. In L. Myers and K. Midence (eds) *Adherence to Treatment*, London: Harwood.

Tones, B.K. and Tilford, S. (1994) *Health Education: Effectiveness, Efficiency and Equity*, 2nd edition, London: Chapman and Hall.

Townsend, J. (1986) Cost effectiveness. In J. Crofton and M. Wood (eds) *Smoking Control: Strategies and Evaluation in Community and Mass Media Programmes*, Report of a workshop, London: Health Education Council.

Vanderplaat, M. (1995) Beyond technique; issues in evaluating for empowerment. *Evaluation*, **1**(1): 81–96.

Warner, M.W. (1994) Present needs and future context: forces for change in health care in the United Kingdom. In K. Lee (ed.) *Health Care Systems in Canada and the United Kingdom*, Keele: Ryburn Publishing.

World Health Organization (1986) *Ottawa Charter for Health Promotion*, Copenhagen: WHO Regional Office for Europe.

Quality assurance programmes: their development and contribution to improving effectiveness in health promotion

5

Viv Speller

The increased interest in quality assurance[1] in health promotion practice, mostly based on methods drawn from the commercial sector, has led to debate about their relevance to health promotion and how they might be applied. The drive to underpin health care purchasing decisions with evidence of effectiveness[2] has also permeated health promotion, resulting in a much sharper focus on evaluating health promotion practice. However, the constructs of 'quality assurance' and 'effective health promotion' and the methodologies involved in their assessment have come to be used synonymously, unhelpfully confusing both the debate and their application in practice.

This chapter seeks to unravel the contributions of quality assurance and effectiveness research to the goal of improving the effectiveness of health promotion and to provide some guidance on developing quality assurance programmes.[3] As will be seen, although the prime responsibility for developing quality assurance programmes lies with health promotion practitioners, researchers of health promotion activity also need to be aware of what constitutes good quality health promotion in designing research studies. The interconnectedness of quality assurance and research into effectiveness and how they may act in combination to improve the effectiveness of health promotion will be discussed.

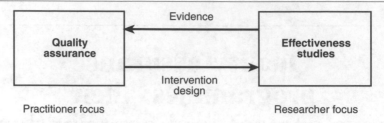

Figure 5.1 Simple relationships between quality assurance and evaluation.

Figure 5.1 presents a very simple model of these relationships. First, we need to distinguish what we mean by 'research' and 'practice' in health promotion and look for the essential links between them that may need development. Here quality assurance is seen as a practitioner focus that should draw upon and integrate research evidence into practice. The research focus of effectiveness reviews is necessary to generate this evidence. Current processes used for systematic reviews of evidence in health care provide a hierarchy of research designs that enable studies to be ranked in relation to the quality of the research. Whilst there is a wider debate about the relevance of these criteria to health promotion research, this chapter will concentrate on the lack of attention paid to the quality of the health promotion interventions assessed. In part this is due to the lack of published consensus about what constitutes quality practice in health promotion, which is a reflection of the current state of the art. Both the links represented by the arrows are fairly weak at the moment and need improving – that from researchers to practitioners by increased access to evidence of effectiveness and that from practitioners to researchers by the recognition that quality criteria[4] need to be applied to the intervention as well as the research process, and by the availability of generalizable standards and criteria.

QUALITY ASSURANCE IN HEALTH PROMOTION

There has been considerable development in quality assurance in health promotion in recent years. Historically, quality assurance in *health education,* particularly in the USA, does not seem to have had any significant influence on the development of quality assurance in the practice of *health promotion.* As early as 1978, Green and Brooks-Bertram described the measurement of quality standards to reflect expected relationships between professional activities and educational outcomes. In 1980, Green recognized the need for the health education profession to set its own standards[5] and criteria for patient education, rather than waiting for other professionals to define appropriate standards for the health education elements of quality assurance programmes in health care. Schwartz (1985) reviewed quality assurance and standards and criteria in health education in the USA, describing a number of examples of quality assurance processes as they applied to patient education, and he reiterated the need for the profession itself to assume leadership for the development of criteria and standards. The central theme of this chapter, that of the distinction between the process evaluation undertaken through quality assurance and the longer term evaluation of the impact of professional activities on client outcomes, was considered by Green and Lewis (1986) who concluded that to assure quality, standards of professional practice need to be applied before effects of programmes are measured. In the following decade there was only patchy progress towards professional consensus of what constitutes quality assurance in health promotion and appropriate evaluation[6] processes, as described below.

The Community Health Accreditation and Standards Project (CHASP) in Australia provides a model for the development of health promotion standards, and encompasses some aspects of health promotion in the community health setting (Fry, 1990). However, again, the aspects covered were mostly only related to educational activities, rather than the breadth of potential health promotion methods. As health education is an integral component of health promotion, these definitions of quality should be nested in the development of quality assurance programmes for the whole range of activities undertaken by health promotion specialists. As Catford (1993) noted, there was a paucity of material on quality assurance for the breadth of health promotion activity. In the UK, the Society of Health Education and Promotion Specialists (SHEPS) produced initial resources in a manual on audit, but included neither measurable standards of practice or a systematic audit process (SHEPS, 1992). The Health Education Authority for England funded a project in 1993 with the aim of providing health promotion practitioners with a theoretical and operational framework within which to address quality assurance. A manual providing guidance on quality assurance concepts and methods, characteristics of good practice in health promotion, model standards *and* criteria and guidance on starting a quality assurance programme was produced and distributed to all health promotion departments in England in 1994 (Evans *et al.*, 1994). The methods and outcomes of this project are detailed elsewhere (Speller *et al.*, 1997a) and key points will be described later in this chapter. Also in 1994, health promotion programme management guidelines were produced in Australia to give practitioners a comprehensive and practical tool for the planning, implementation and maintenance of health promotion programmes (Central Sydney Area Health Service and NSW Health, 1994).

Subsequently, Simnett (1995) and Ovretveit (1996) have described the relationship between quality assurance and health promotion, placing emphasis on three dimensions of quality practice for health promotion: *management quality*,[7] *professional quality*[8] and *consumer quality*[9] or participation by local people. While the congruence between these quality methods and health promotion practice is acknowledged, neither provides practical guidance or transferable standards of health promotion practice.

It may be helpful to distinguish between attempts to generate processes and/or lists of standards for *quality assurance programmes*, that aim in an organized way to ensure the quality of the total range of health promotion programmes provided by a health promotion service, *and* the approach to develop *quality initiatives*[10] in particular settings, where standards are agreed with the relevant stakeholders and applied to the design and implementation of an intervention. Quality assessment procedures have been described for work place health promotion (Lowe *et al.*, 1989; Kizer *et al.*, 1992); for particular types of educational interventions such as peer education (Croll *et al.*, 1993); and for healthy alliances (Funnell *et al.*, 1995). In the Wessex Institute for Health Research and Development, we have developed a number of quality initiatives, which have built in external as well as internal accreditation processes and which may lead to a recognized 'award'. For example, the Wessex Healthy Schools Award was developed in 1993 and has accredited over 300 schools in the south of England, some of which are now entering their third year of revalidation (Rogers *et al.*, 1993). This scheme aims to develop 'health-promoting schools', through audit of current status, identification of areas for change and assessment of progress. It encompasses nine key areas of activity, each with agreed standards and indicators of achievement. The Healthy Leisure Award was developed in a similar multidisciplinary manner with health and leisure providers and launched in 1996. Centres are assessed by an independent assessor against eight key statements, target areas for improvement are agreed and a portfolio of progress kept for subsequent reassessment to achieve the award (Wessex Institute, 1996). Similarly, an organizational audit[11] framework has been developed to help implement the concept of the health-promoting hospital. The audit framework consists of eight elements embracing existing quality approaches in the acute setting as well as their role in promoting health; audit is by self-assessment and peer review (Rushmere and Kickham, 1998).

The European Commission sponsored a project in 1996 to review quality assessment and health promotion intervention evaluation in the 15 member states. Fourteen took part, providing the first survey in the EU on quality assurance and evaluation in health promotion (IUHPE/EURO, 1996). This identified a continuing confusion, both in terminology, and between attention to quality assurance processes for the planning and implementation stages of a programme versus effect evaluation. Many countries cited examples of outcome indicators used to judge changes in health behaviour and health as a result of health promotion programmes, rather than quality assurance standards and criteria. However, the review identified some other interesting examples of measurement tools or instruments and there was a degree of consensus on some fundamental issues surrounding quality assurance and evaluation emerging from the workshop discussions in which all the national teams took part. A consensus definition was reached: 'Quality assurance in health promotion is the process of assessment of a programme or intervention in order to ensure performance against agreed standards, which are subject to continuous improvement and set within the framework and principles of the Ottawa Charter'.

In Belgium, explicit criteria are used for the planning of health promotion interventions; projects must conform to these when applying for government funding (Lievens and van den Broucke, 1995). In Sweden, a manual and guidance have been produced for practitioners to help them in the quality assurance of structure, process and outcome of health promotion projects (Socialstyrelsen, 1995; Landstingsforbundet, 1996) and in The Netherlands there is an instrument for assessing the development of health education leaflets, videos and new media (Saan, 1996). The Netherlands have also produced a tool for the planning and evaluation of health promotion interventions, the Health Promotion Effectiveness Fostering Instrument (PREFFI). This is intended to be used alongside a similar tool for researchers assessing effectiveness through systematic reviews of the literature, ANALYS (Keijsers et al., 1996). This is an interesting example of an approach for linking quality assessment in both practice and research. Before considering these links further, it is necessary to look closely at the lessons learnt from the UK experience of developing quality assurance in health promotion.

DEVELOPING QUALITY ASSURANCE PROGRAMMES IN HEALTH PROMOTION TEAMS

The manual *Assuring Quality in Health Promotion* (Evans et al., 1994) considered four key aspects of quality assurance programmes: the quality assurance cycle; identification of key functions of health promotion; the need for a 'quality culture' and ownership of quality assurance processes by teams; and consideration of assessment methods.

Quality assurance cycle

In order to emphasize the developmental aspects of the process of quality assurance, the definition chosen for the project was adapted from Wright and Whittington (1992): 'Quality assurance is a systematic process

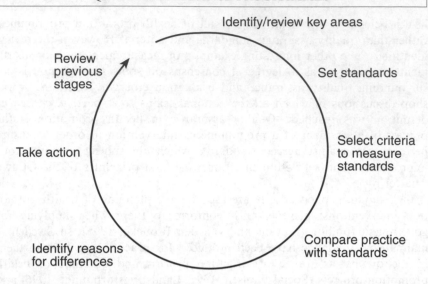

Figure 5.2   The quality assurance cycle. From Evans *et al.*, 1994. Copyright ©
1994, Health Education Authority. Reproduced with permission.

through which achievable and desirable levels of quality are described, the
extent to which these levels are achieved is assessed, and action is taken
following assessment to enable them to be reached'. This process is
described as a six-stage cycle (Ellis and Whittington, 1993) and the project
provided advice and tools for approaching each stage of the cycle (Figure
5.2). *Standards* were described as: 'statements defining agreed levels of
excellence of performance that should be acceptable to colleagues and
service users'. *Criteria* were defined as: 'descriptive statements which are
measurable that are used to assess the level of performance towards
meeting the standard'.

Key functions of health promotion

In order to derive measurable standards and criteria to assess the quality
of the diversity of health promotion practice, it was necessary to break it
down into discrete 'chunks' of activity that were clearly recognizable as
important core functions of health promotion, although individually they
may also be aspects of the work of other professionals. However, the sum
of these aspects, or key functions, needs to encompass the full breadth of
practice that health promotion specialists undertake. The World Health
Organization's definition of health promotion, as a process of enabling
people to increase control over and to improve their health (WHO, 1984),

and the Ottawa Charter (WHO, 1986) are widely accepted as the aims and principles of health promotion practice but are difficult to operationalize in terms of the specific actions that health promoters take towards these goals. The relative value of deriving standards for specific settings, methods or health topics was considered but as services are organized differently according to local health priorities and the skills of practitioners, it was felt a more generic set of standards that reflected the functional processes of health promotion practice would be more appropriate. Six key functions were identified as a result: strategic planning, programme management, monitoring[12] and evaluation, education and training, resources and information, and advice and consultancy. The first three reflect the principles of identifying need, setting objectives, designing action plans and managing programmes of work to meet them and assessing the extent to which objectives have been met. These are essentially the management steps underlying the provision of any high quality service and are as relevant to health promotion activity as to any other. The latter three describe the major ways in which health promotion specialists work in order to achieve their goals. These key functions could be applied to different programme areas, such as heart disease prevention, smoking cessation or HIV/AIDS; or age groups, such as young people, or settings, such as schools, primary care or the work place. A quality assurance programme therefore could be organized by assessing each of the key functions horizontally in relation to a particular programme area, or vertically, by assessing the quality of individual key functions such as programme management or education and training, across all the health promotion programmes in a department.

Twenty-five model standards were agreed (3–6 for each key function) and 106 criteria derived (2–7 for each standard) by which to assess progress towards the standards. The standards are listed in Table 5.1. The criteria underlying the standards provide more detail about the expectations implicit in the standard statement and measurable steps or indicators of its achievement.

Developing a 'quality assurance culture' in health promotion teams

However, it was recognized that these generic standards were a starting point and that it would be necessary to tailor them to local circumstances and develop them with experience of their application. Therefore guidance on the ways to adapt them or to develop additional local standards was also provided. Practitioners indicated that they needed support in developing an understanding of quality assurance processes within their teams, as well as practical suggestions for implementing a quality assurance programme. The project devised a number of group exercises to lead team members into this process, by considering issues such as what constitutes

Table 5.1 Model standards for each of the key functions

	Standards	
1. Strategic planning	1.1	There is a group which addresses strategic planning issues in health promotion
	1.2	The health promotion service makes an important contribution to this group
	1.3	A health promotion strategy is produced and/or health promotion figures prominently within other health strategy documents
	1.4	The health promotion department's plan relates to the health strategies
2. Programme management	2.1	A group exists for the planning, implementation and review of each programme area
	2.2	A range of health promotion methods and activities is considered for each programme area in order to determine action plans
	2.3	For each programme a health promotion specialist is identified who is competent to lead
	2.4	Arrangements are made for reporting on progress
3. Monitoring and evaluation	3.1	There are agreed arrangements for monitoring and evaluation of all programmes
	3.2	The results of programme evaluation are used to inform further work
	3.3	Support is given to members of staff to develop their skills with regard to monitoring and evaluation
4. Education and training	4.1	An education and training plan exists for the health promotion department
	4.2	Training programmes are based upon the results of needs assessment with client groups
	4.3	All training includes an evaluation exercise
	4.4	Training is provided by qualified and experienced trainers
	4.5	Administrative procedures ensure that the training programme is delivered efficiently
5. Resources and information	5.1	The provider has a resources and information plan as part of its health promotion strategy or business plan
	5.2	There is a procedure for reviewing resources and information held
	5.3	The services available are widely advertised for optimal uptake by existing and potential clients
	5.4	Clients feel valued and welcome when they visit the department
	5.5	Resources and information services are adequately housed
	5.6	Clients' views of services are regularly sought and acted upon
6. Advice and consultancy	6.1	Staff function within the SHEPS Principles of Practice and Code of Conduct (or equivalent)
	6.2	Advice given is based upon the elicited and expressed needs of clients
	6.3	Confidentiality is maintained at all times with regard to personal information about clients
	6.4	Staff are competent in those aspects of health promotion in which advice is given
	6.5	All staff with an advisory role receive training in communication skills

good practice, the extent to which theoretical definitions of good practice are applied in the work setting and what quality assurance means to individuals. Given the diverse nature of health promotion activity and the varied experience and skills of health promotion specialists, a range of opinions about the relative merits of different approaches exists within the profession as a whole and within teams. The purpose of reflection on the definitions of quality practice is not to determine which approach may be more valid but to acknowledge the philosophical differences and, crucially, to recognize that quality assurance applies to all types of health promotion activity and that they are all amenable to systematic review. It was clear that working through these group exercises helped practitioners to articulate their concerns about the introduction of quality assurance and enabled them to arrive at a consensus about how to take the process forward in their own work.

Assessment methods

The assessment[13] stage of the quality assurance cycle is fundamental to the process. Criteria need to have been described so as to be measurable, but assessment methods need to be planned and agreed at the outset, so that it is clear to all parties what is expected and sufficient resources are available to undertake the review stage. An assessment protocol was derived allowing for identification of assessor, assessment method, a five-point achievement code and proforma for documenting priorities for further development resulting from review.

Two years after dissemination, progress in implementing quality assurance in health promotion departments based upon the guidance provided in the manual was reviewed. Problems perceived included a persisting confusion over terminology, operational issues such as time and pressures of organizational change and feeling threatened by the possibility of quality assurance becoming another management tool. There were concerns that purchasers might take greater control of quality assurance and emphasize inappropriate measures, or might constrain flexibility of action through too much formalization of the process. On the positive side, practitioners valued having a framework to structure work and define philosophy and there were benefits to internal communications and staff development. The importance of quality assurance in external relations was also seen to be important through helping to raise the profile of the service and to meet purchasers' contract requirements. When practitioners were asked to consider the future direction of quality assurance and support requirements, there were clear concerns about the relationship between quality and effectiveness. In particular, practitioners still found difficulty in differentiating between process, impact and outcome measurement. Practitioners identified that further support was required in training and development to implement quality assurance processes and in access to evidence of effectiveness.

RELATIONSHIPS BETWEEN QUALITY ASSURANCE AND RESEARCH FOR EFFECTIVE HEALTH PROMOTION

Returning to the simple model presented in Figure 5.1, we have seen how health promotion practitioners are developing and using skills in quality assurance processes to improve the standards of health promotion practice and how limitations on access to evidence of effectiveness are highlighted as a constraint in developing effective practice. On the research side of the equation we have an increasing supply of such information in systematic reviews of effectiveness in health promotion which are being disseminated to practitioners by, for example, the Health Education Authority. However, the limitations of the review process as it is applied to health promotion are becoming clearer, as are deficiencies in primary research into health promotion, with consequent concerns about its potential negative impact on the future of health promotion (Speller *et al.*, 1997b). Nutbeam (1996) considered a number of ways in which the fit between research and practice could be improved: through improving communication between researchers and practitioners; influencing funding bodies to support relevant research; encouraging researchers to report on findings in ways accessible to practitioners and policymakers; and improving practitioner education and training. He presented a sequential model of the relationship between different types of research and their relevance to practitioners which demonstrates that research into problem definition is dominant in volume terms but is of least significance to practice.

By contrast, research into testing solutions, i.e. health promotion interventions, is less common but is crucial to the advancement of effective health promotion. Interestingly, Nutbeam places quality control at the bottom of the hierarchy of research types but, with its expected outcomes of maintenance of conditions for success and monitoring of effects, of most usefulness and relevance to practitioners. Macdonald (1996) also debates the future of evaluation in health promotion and cites four key principles of the philosophical base of health promotion evaluative research: using needs assessment methods; espousing user involvement; applying quality assurance procedures in relation to the appropriateness of the intervention; and respect for the use of both audit and evaluation methods. It is the contention of this chapter that quality assurance principles and methods need to be more centrally engaged in the process of evaluating health promotion than hitherto. The domains of research and practice are still too separate and the debate tends to focus on the failings of practitioners to understand or use evidence when it becomes available.

Responsibility also rests with the research community to understand and learn from the practice of health promotion; the call for far greater involvement of policymakers and practitioners in the planning and conduct of research (Green and Kok, 1990) is still rarely heeded.

If we wish to understand the effects of health promotion interventions, detailed research studies are required. In order to analyse the steps necessary to move from hypothesis to routine practice and the contribution that quality assurance makes along this route, we need to consider an 'ideal' process of research. The model presented in Figure 5.3 summarizes key steps in the research process and identifies the contribution of quality assurance. The sequence of steps is adapted from the eight-stage model for phases of health promotion research described by Flay (1986). He proposed that basic research on the causal mechanisms of health would lead to hypothesis development about new approaches to health promotion for a specific health problem. Preliminary tests of new approaches would be piloted, leading to small-scale prototype studies of further refined programmes. These would then be tested for their efficacy in efficacy trials to determine whether the programme or intervention does more good than harm when delivered under optimum conditions of implementation and compliance by the target group. This stage is often not included in health promotion research but without it, it is difficult to assess whether negative results of a programme are due to the way in which a programme was implemented or whether it was inefficacious. Flay then considers two types of effectiveness trials, which assess whether a treatment does more good than harm in 'real-world' conditions. First, he contends that implementation processes should be controlled, allowing for study of the acceptability of the programme, and thereafter the implementation is allowed to vary to assess implementation effectiveness. Finally, demonstration studies of an efficacious and effective programme would be studied on a large scale in whole communities to assess the overall impact on public health. Such a rigorous and systematic process of evaluation is rarely if ever conducted and so the model in Figure 5.3 attempts to clarify the essential steps and draw upon routine practice in order to render the whole more achievable.

The first stage of intervention development is informed by the empirical and theoretical basis of the health issue in question and hypotheses of the effect of interventions. This requires knowledge of evidence of methodological effects, but to optimize the design, theory needs to be augmented by professional and community views to ensure appropriateness and acceptability. Thus this is congruent with Ovretveit's (1996) concepts of professional and consumer quality. In the design stage, small-scale pilots testing consensus with groups of stakeholders are vital. This is similar to the quality assurance cycle in that, with each phase of testing and review, performance against standards set will be assessed and adjusted. In the

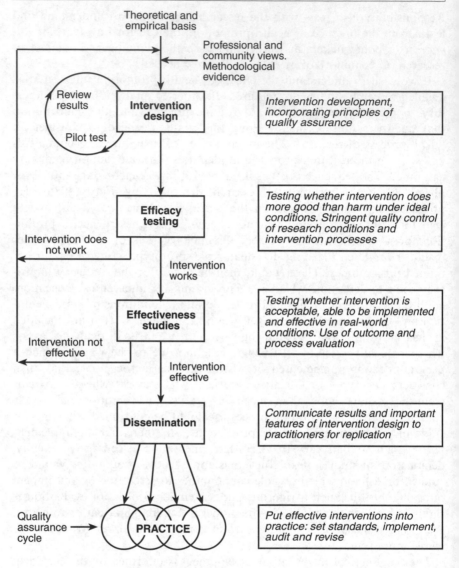

Figure 5.3 Relationships between quality assurance and stages in research into effectiveness of health promotion interventions.

development phases of the Healthy Schools Award and Healthy Leisure Award described above, lengthy iterative processes were undertaken to ensure that the intervention design was optimized, was acceptable and, within the limits of piloting, was able to be put into practice as expected.

The second phase of efficacy testing is rarely undertaken, often due to financial constraints and the pressure to disseminate an intervention as widely as possible. This requires stringent quality control of both the research conditions and the intervention processes. In order to control these conditions it is necessary to have explicit standards of all aspects of the intervention and to rigorously monitor these throughout the research to ensure compliance with procedures. If the intervention does not have the anticipated outcomes, a return to the previous design stage is required in order to assess whether there are improvements to the intervention that can be made or whether there are faults regarding the underlying theory and causal mechanisms. If it is efficacious, it is then possible to proceed to the next stage of effectiveness testing. Here the intervention is tested in real-world situations, with an attempt to optimize performance through, for example, training of personnel involved. However, variations will naturally occur in the way the intervention is undertaken and in other factors influencing the target group. Exposure to the media, for example, or diffusion of effects through communities cannot be controlled. Process evaluation of the intervention is necessary to check on the match between intended and actual implementation, to understand how acceptable the intervention is to the target group and illuminate other influences on their behaviour.

The Wessex Healthy Schools Award is now the subject of a quasi-experimental controlled trial to evaluate its effect both on the health behaviour and knowledge of pupils and on policies and practices within the schools. The research design incorporates both qualitative and quantitative evaluation methods and assesses impact from a variety of perspectives. In an ideal world, this would have been conducted prior to its wider implementation. Only if the intervention is effective should it be disseminated into practice, but there are often perverse incentives in the system not to do this. In this case the high visibility, penetration and perceived success of the programme rendered it acceptable to funders for evaluation. Many health promotion programmes are marketed or put into practice without evidence of effect and conversely, results of research studies may only be published in academic journals and little attention is paid to their wider dissemination to the practice community, as Nutbeam (1996) describes. Given the lack of attention in many research studies to process evaluation, important features of the intervention design may not be known or not disseminated, thereby reducing the ability of practitioners to adopt the methods, as in the final stage of this model. Here practitioners put effective programmes into practice and maintain their impact through quality assurance procedures, as described previously. Within a framework of agreed standards, local modifications and levels of performance can be agreed according to resource limits and monitored to ensure compliance.

Quality assurance and effectiveness research in health promotion are not therefore separate endeavours, but are interwoven in an ideal process of intervention testing and delivery. Health promotion practitioners have a central part to play in the design of interventions for testing, in particular to ensure that issues relating to consumer perceptions of quality have been considered which will maximize acceptability and professional views are built in, primarily to ensure that implementation is feasible. In the testing phases, their contribution is essential to maintain the standards of the intervention, through training, support and facilitation for the health promotion programme, within the evaluative framework designed by the researchers. Researchers and practitioners need to come together to learn from the experience of research studies and not only for practitioners to passively receive data, but to assist with its interpretation and with the logistics of wider replication. At this point the clarification of key success features identified through both outcome and process evaluation will form the basis for setting implementation standards for practice, which will be sustained through routine quality assurance programmes.

NOTES

1. Quality assurance – the systematic process through which achievable and desirable levels of quality are described, the extent to which these levels are achieved is assessed, and action is taken following assessment to enable them to be reached (Evans *et al.*, 1994).
2. Effectiveness – whether a technology, treatment, procedure, intervention or programme does more good than harm when delivered under real-world conditions (Flay, 1986).
3. Quality assurance programme – programmes that aim in an organized way to ensure the quality of the total range of health promotion programmes provided by a health promotion service.
4. Criteria – descriptive statements which are measurable, that relate to a standard. Sometimes the term 'indicator' is used synonymously (Evans *et al.*, 1994; IUHPE/EURO, 1996).
5. Standard – a statement which defines an agreed level of excellence (Evans *et al.*, 1994); agreed level of service or practice (IUHPE/EURO, 1996).
6. Evaluation – this is concerned with assessing or measuring an activity against predetermined goals or values (IUHPE/EURO, 1996).
7. Management quality – whether the programme is planned, designed and provided or implemented in a way which makes best use of resources, without waste or mistakes, and which meets higher level requirements (as measured by the costs of poor quality and in relation to policies and targets set by higher levels) (Ovretveit, 1996).
8. Professional quality – whether the programme meets individual and community needs for health promotion as assessed by health promotion professionals; and whether the programme is designed and provided in a way which professionals believe will prevent illness and promote health (as measured by different

professional assessments of the programme and by outcome indicators and long-term measures) (Ovretveit, 1996).

9. Consumer quality – whether the programme gives individuals and the community what they say they want to help them prevent illness and improve health (as measured by people's satisfaction with health promotion and health education programmes) (Ovretveit, 1996).

10. Quality initiative – this applies to particular health promotion settings or interventions, where standards are derived with the relevant stakeholders and applied to the design and implementation of a specific intervention.

11. Audit – the systematic critical analysis of the quality of a health promotion programme, considered to be synonymous with quality assurance. Sometimes used to describe the review stage in a quality assurance process (Evans *et al.*, 1994; IUHPE/EURO, 1996).

12. Monitoring – the process of collecting and analysing information about programme evaluation over time to ensure planned activities are carried out and problems are identified (Evans *et al.*, 1994; IUHPE/EURO, 1996).

13. Quality assessment – the process of assessment of a programme or intervention in order to ensure performance against agreed standards, which are subject to continuous improvement and set within the framework and principles of the Ottawa Charter (IUHPE/EURO, 1996).

REFERENCES

Catford, J. (1993) Auditing health promotion: what are the vital signs of quality? *Health Promotion International*, **8**(2), 67–68.

Central Sydney Area Health Service and NSW Health. (1994) *Program Management Guidelines for Health Promotion*, New South Wales State Health Publication (HP) 94-143.

Croll, N., Jurs, E. and Kennedy, S. (1993) Total quality assurance and peer education. *Journal of the American College of Health*, **41**(6), 247–249.

Ellis, R. and Whittington, D. (1993) *Quality Assurance in Health Care: A Handbook*, London: Edward Arnold.

Evans, D., Head, D. and Speller, V. (1994) *Assuring Quality in Health Promotion: How to Develop Standards of Good Practice*, London: Health Education Authority.

Flay, B.R. (1986) Efficacy and effectiveness trials (and other phases of research) in the development of health promotion programs. *Preventive Medicine*, **15**, 451–474.

Fry, D. (1990) Systems of standards for community health services in Australia. *Quality Assurance in Health Care*, **2**, 59–67.

Funnell, R., Oldfield, K. and Speller, V. (1995) *Towards Healthier Alliances, a Tool for Planning, Evaluating and Developing Healthy Alliances*, London: Health Education Authority.

Green, L.W. (1980) What is quality in patient education and how do we assess it? In W. Squires (ed.) *Patient Education: An Enquiry into the State of the Art*, New York: Springer.

Green, L.W. and Brooks-Bertram, P. (1978) Peer review and quality control in health education. In: *Health values achieving high level wellness.* **2**(4), 191–197.

Green, L.W. and Kok, G. (1990) Research to support health promotion in practice: a plea for increased co-operation. *Health Promotion International*, **5**, 303–308.

Green, L.W. and Lewis, F.M. (1986) *Measurement and Evaluation in Health Education and Health Promotion*, Palo Alto, CA: Mayfield.

IUHPE/EURO (1996) *Presentation of Existing Standards for Evaluation and Quality Assessment of Health Promotion Interventions in the EU Member States 1996*, Woerden:, IUHPE Regional Office for Europe.

Keijsers, J.F.E.M., Molleman, G.M.R. and van Driel, W.G. (1996) Reviewing and guiding the effectiveness of behavioural health promotion. Paper presented at 3rd IUHPE European Conference of Effectiveness. Quality Assessment in Health Promotion and Health Education, Turin, Italy.

Kizer, K.W., Folkers, L.F., Felten, P.G and Neimeyer, D. (1992) Quality assessment in worksite health promotion. *American Journal of Preventive Medicine*, **8**(2), 123–127.

Landstingsforbundet (1996) *Succeeding with Health Promotion Projects – Quality Assurance*, Stockholm: Landstingsforbundet.

Lievens, P. and van den Broucke, S. (1995) Strategic planning for health promotion: the Flemish experience. *Promotion and Education*, **2**, 91–97.

Lowe, J.B., Windsor, R.A. and Valois, R.F. (1989) Quality assurance methods for managing employee health promotion programs: a case study in smoking cessation. *Health Values*, **13**(2), 17–23.

Macdonald, G. (1996) Where next for evaluation? *Health Promotion International*, **11**, 171–173.

Nutbeam, D. (1996) Achieving 'best practice' in health promotion: improving the fit between research and practice. *Health Promotion International*, **11**, 317–326.

Ovretveit, J. (1996) Quality in health promotion. *Health Promotion International*, **11**(1), 55–62.

Roger, E., Taylor, P. and Gott, D. (1993) *The Wessex Healthy Schools Award*, Winchester: Wessex Institute for Public Health Medicine.

Rushmere, A. and Kickham, N. (1998) Alliances in secondary care: health promoting hospitals. In A. Scriven (ed.) *Healthy Alliances in Theory and Practice*, London: Macmillan.

Saan, J.A.M. (1996) Voorstel Kwaliteitscriteria. Video en brochures, Woerden: NIGZ.

Schwartz, R. (1985) Quality assurance, standards and criteria in health education: a review. *Patient Education and Counselling*, **7**, 325–335.

Simnett, I. (1995) *Managing Health Promotion; Developing Healthy Organisations and Communities*, Chichester: John Wiley.

Socialstyrelsen (1995) *Kvalitet I forebyggande och halsoframjande arbete*, Stockholm: Socialstyrelsen.

Society of Health Education and Health Promotion Specialists (1992) *Developing Quality in Health Education and Health Promotion*, SHEPS.

Speller, V., Evans, D. and Head, M. (1997a) Developing quality assurance standards for health promotion practice in the UK. *Health Promotion International*, **12**(3), 215–224.

Speller, V., Learmonth, A. and Harrison, D. (1997b) The search for evidence of effective health promotion. *British Medical Journal*, **315**, 361–363.

Wessex Institute for Health Research and Development (1996) *Healthy Leisure Award Portfolio*, Southampton: University of Southampton.

World Health Organization (1984) *Health Promotion: a WHO Document on the Concepts and Principles*, Copenhagen: WHO.

World Health Organization (1986) *The Ottawa Charter, Principles for Health Promotion*, Copenhagen: WHO Regional Office for Europe.

Wright, C. and Whittington, D. (1992) *Quality Assurance: an Introduction for Health Care Professionals*, Edinburgh: Churchill Livingstone.

<table>
| 6 | **Planning and evaluating health promotion** |
</table>

Hein De Vries

With regard to health education and health promotion, various definitions, interpretations and models exist. One common theme, however, is that all the strategies focus on stimulating the adoption of healthy behaviours among individuals or groups of individuals. Another important common theme relates to the fact that the chances for effective health education and promotion will increase if they are systematic and planned undertakings (Kok and De Vries, 1989; Green and Kreuter, 1991; Tones and Tilford, 1994).

The goal of this chapter is to present a comprehensive model for planning health education and promotion that integrates principles of planning with psychological principles about motivational change. The planning model is the result of the integration of several planning models that have been used in the field of health education and applied psychology, most notably the Precede-Proceed model for health education and promotion (Green and Kreuter, 1991), the Community Change Model (Bracht, 1990), theories about behavioural change (McGuire, 1985) and theories about diffusion (Rogers, 1995). I will furthermore describe some practical tools that can be used to facilitate the application of theory to practice.

HEALTH PROMOTION AND MOTIVATION

An important feature of health promotion is that it is aimed at motivating (groups of) individuals to adopt healthy behaviours. Various descriptions of a healthy behaviour can be given. We will refer to a healthy behaviour as an action of individuals, organizations or institutions that is conducive to their or others' health. This description embraces both individual health behaviours (i.e. non-smoking) as well as social health behaviours, such as the development and implementation of health-promoting policies (i.e. stimulating general practitioners to give smoking cessation education to their patients). This definition also implies that target groups can be selected at the individual or micro level, the social or meso level or the institutional or macro level and that at each level, the goal is to stimulate the target group to adopt healthy behaviours.

A distinction can be made between three main types of models for health promotion. The first type concerns planning models. They are aimed at guiding practitioners and researchers through the process of the planning of health promotion activities and research by identifying main phases, which sometimes are further divided into planning steps. A second type concerns explanatory models which intend to describe why people adopt a particular (health) behaviour. A third type concerns change theories which discuss how we can stimulate behavioural change. While the main focus of this chapter is on discussion of a planning strategy, I will also briefly summarize some important explanatory and change models when describing planning steps.

PLANNING MODELS

A prerequisite for effective health promotion activities is that they are undertaken systematically. A systematic approach is facilitated by the utilization of a health promotion planning model. A planning model serves to identify important phases (and steps within these phases) in order to plan ahead and make sound decisions. The advantage of using a planning model is that many relevant aspects are dealt with systematically, that it provides an overview of the main issues that need attention and that it can serve as a checklist during the process of planning. A planning model stimulates practitioners to plan ahead and may prevent the development of ineffective programmes (Kok and De Vries, 1989; Kok and Green, 1990).Various health promotion planning models have been developed. I will describe the main models and will conclude with an indepth discussion of an integrative planning model.

Precede-Proceed Model

In 1980, Green and colleagues described the PRECEDE model for health education planning (Green et al., 1980). This model distinguishes five phases in the planning of health education strategies. It states that health education should start with a social diagnosis to determine people's perceptions of their own needs or quality of life and their aspirations for the common good (Green and Kreuter, 1991). The second phase is the epidemiological diagnosis to determine which health problems are important. In the behavioural and environmental diagnosis, the third phase, the main determinants of the health problem are analysed. This is followed by a diagnosis of the relevant educational and organizational factors, in which an analysis is made of the predisposing, reinforcing and enabling factors that need to be changed to initiate and sustain a process of behavioural and environmental change. These factors will become the immediate targets of a health promotion programme. The fifth phase is the administrative and policy diagnosis and focuses on developing health education and health regulation actions.

In 1991, the PRECEDE model was elaborated with a PROCEDE part, describing the process that occurred after the development of health promotion interventions. This added: evaluations of the implementation of the actions (phase 6), the effects of these actions on the predisposing, reinforcing and enabling factors (phase 7), the changes in the behaviours of individuals and in the environment (phase 8), and the outcomes of the health promotion actions on health and the quality of life (phase 9).

The Community Organization Stage Model

This model (Bracht, 1990; Bracht and Kingsbury, 1990) distinguishes five stages for the development of community programmes. The first stage of the model is the analysis of the community to obtain information about its needs, resources, social structure and values. Another goal of this phase is to identify citizen leaders and the extent of organizational involvement to create collaborative and broad community participation. The second stage concerns the development of the design of the community programme and the initiation of the development of an organizational structure and the preparation of plans. The third phase focuses on implementing those plans. The fourth stage looks at programme maintenance and consolidation. During this stage, community members and staff gain experience and success with the programme and the problems that arose at the beginning of the project have now been dealt with. The final stage addresses the dissemination of the programme and the reassessment of activities. In this phase, the community analysis is updated, the effectiveness of interventions is established and future directions and modifications are discussed.

Diffusion theory

Diffusion theory is not a planning model but has been used to guide health promotion planning. Health promotion programmes can be considered as innovations for many groups and therefore Rogers' theory of diffusion of innovations has been used to understand the adoption process of health promotion programmes. Diffusion is defined as the process by which an innovation is communicated through certain channels over time among the members of a social system. Rogers (1995:11) defines an innovation as 'an idea, practice or object that is perceived as new by an individual or other unit of adoption'. Rogers also indicates that the chances of successful adoption are determined by various characteristics of the innovation, such as the relative advantages and its compatibility.

An important notion from the diffusion theory for health promotion is that the adoption of health promotion programmes can occur at different rates. Groups differ in their rate of adoption resulting in populations of innovators, early adopters, the early majority, the late majority and laggards. Consequently, different marketing strategies for these groups may be needed to convince them to use a particular programme.

Other planning models

Other planning models have been formulated, such as PATCH, a variation on the PRECEDE model (Kreuter, 1992), the Model for Management of Intervention Programme Preparation (MMIPP) (Sanderson *et al.*, 1996) and the ONPRIME model (Elder *et al.*, 1994). Instead of debating the best way of describing the various stages, I propose to look at the similarities of the different planning models.

One important observation is that three main phases can be distinguished. The first is a preparatory phase (formative evaluation): the actions that are needed to prepare a programme. A second phase is programme development, implementation and testing. A third phase is programme diffusion.

Another commonality is the absence of clear applications of motivational principles with regard to health promotion planning activities. I will therefore describe a model integrating principles about planning and motivation which will be illustrated with practical tools to enhance its application.

THE ABC PLANNING MODEL

The ABC model for planning motivational change (De Vries, 1989; 1991; Dijkstra *et al.*, 1993) distinguishes three basic phases: analysing the problem; behavioural change; and continuation of prevention (Figure 6.1).

Analysis of the problem

Within the analysis phase, five steps are identified: needs assessment; the analysis of factors concerning health problems; the selection of target groups; the analysis of motivational factors; and access points analysis.

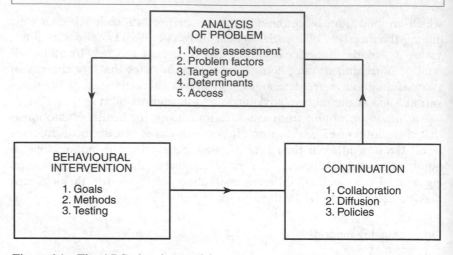

Figure 6.1   The ABC planning model.

Needs assessment

This phase addresses issues such as the quality of life and the physical, mental and health problems of a particular population of interest. Examples of physical problems are cardiovascular diseases, cancer, asthma and diabetes. Examples of psychological problems are depression and work stress. Examples of social problems are unemployment, vandalism and crime. Groups within a community may differ with regard to the recognition of a problem and, consequently, their willingness to change a problem. For instance, managers of work sites may want to improve safety regulations, but their employees do not encounter any problems with respect to their safety. Generating consensus on the priorities among various stakeholders is therefore important in order to generate involvement of all the relevant groups. The goal of this phase is to select a particular health problem that requires attention and to generate consensus and interest.

Problem factors

The second phase is the analysis of factors relating to a particular health problem. Two different types of problem factors can be distinguished: individual and external. Individual factors refer to biological factors (e.g. gender, age, type of skin) and psychological factors (e.g. motivation, knowledge). External factors comprise physical factors such as social, geographical and cultural factors (e.g. school regulations, community norms, national laws). The goal of this phase is to select a particular problem factor and the risk behaviour (e.g. smoking, unprotected sunbathing) related to it as well as the recommended health behaviour (e.g. non-smoking, use of sun screen).

Identification of the target group

After the selection of a particular problem factor it is important to identify the target group. This phase is not explicitly mentioned in many planning models. Three different levels of target groups can be distinguished (Tones and Tilford, 1994). The individual or micro level refers to (groups of) individuals who are performing a particular risk behaviour. The meso or social level consists of social settings which often have a direct impact on individuals, such as families, schools and work sites. The macro or institutional level consists of community and national institutions responsible for developing policies and creating facilities. For example, when trying to reduce the impact of smoking, workers at the work site could be chosen as the target group at the individual level, the management at work sites could be chosen as the meso level target group to realize non-smoking policies, while the government could be the target group at the macro level for developing national non-smoking laws for work places. This phase therefore aims at identifying the target groups at the three levels and at specifying clearly the corresponding health behaviours.

Motivational determinants

The fourth phase is to analyse why a target group engages in a particular unhealthy behaviour. Various social psychological models (some are briefly summarized below) suggest that healthy behaviour is determined by a person's motivation (or intention) to perform the behaviour, provided that they are capable of realizing their intention and are not hindered by barriers. Intentions are determined by three types of motivational factors: attitudes, social encouragement and self-efficacy expectations. Attitudes refer to a person's overall evaluation of the behaviour, which is determined by the weighing of the perceived advantages and disadvantages of the behaviour. Social encouragement is determined by perceptions of social norms (opinions of others about the healthy behaviour), social modelling (healthy behaviours of others) and actual social support from others to perform the behaviour. Self-efficacy refers to a person's expectation that they will be able to realize the desired healthy behaviour. Although the references to these concepts differ for each theoretical model, many social-psychological models have included these cognitive determinants, such as Social Learning Theory (Bandura, 1986), the Health Belief Model (Janz and Becker, 1984), Theory of Reasoned Action (Ajzen and Fishbein, 1980), Theory of Planned Behaviour (Ajzen, 1988), the Transtheoretical Model (Prochaska and DiClemente, 1983; Prochaska et al., 1994) and the

Attitude-Social Influence-Efficacy (or ASE) Model (De Vries *et al.*, 1988; De Vries and Mudde, 1997). In summary, the goal of this phase is to analyse whether a target group is convinced of the advantages of the healthy behaviour, receives sufficient social encouragement and has high self-efficacy expectations, and to formulate recommendations about the goals that should be accomplished to create a more positive motivation for adopting particular healthy behaviours.

Access point analysis

The fifth phase concentrates on analysing how the target group can be reached. This implies a careful analysis of the target group's preference for particular methods, the ways to access the target group (e.g. through schools), as well as preferences of programme providers and, finally, research describing effective methods.The goal of this phase is to formulate recommendations about effective methods that will be acceptable for the target group and the programme providers.

Behavioural change

The goal of this phase is to formulate the programme goals, to implement the programme and to assess its efficacy.

Goals

The results of the analysis phase will provide the essential ingredients to formulate goals and select methods. Three types of goals can be distinguished. Programme goals describe the focus of the programme (primary, secondary or tertiary prevention), the target group and the expected effects of the programme within a specific period of time. For instance, 'The programme's goal is to prevent youngsters of 12–14 years taking up smoking, resulting in a 10% lower rate of new smokers after one year'. Method goals refer to the ways the target group will be reached by describing the approach that will be chosen (i.e. education, policies or both), the strategies that will be used (e.g. persuasion, training of skills), access points (e.g. schools, youth clubs) and the channels to be used (e.g. videos, cartoons). Timetable goals describe how the various activities need to be accomplished in time and by whom. It is also important to monitor whether a consensus exists among the stakeholders regarding these goals, for instance by performing process evaluations.

Programme development

When developing a programme, it is important to acknowledge that it should address three distinct phases in the behavioural change process of the target group: reception of information; processing of information; and behavioural actions. Furthermore, the effectiveness of information is determined by receiver factors, message factors, channel factors and source factors (McGuire, 1985). Receiver factors refer to the characteristics of the target group that may influence information processing (e.g. knowledge, motivational stage, educational level). Message factors describe the characteristics of effective messages (e.g. moderate levels of discrepancy between the message and the target group's opinion, utilization of explicit conclusions, repetition of messages). Channel factors refer to the methods by which messages are delivered (e.g. videos, schools). Source factors refer to the characteristics of the persons who provide the programme and the messages. Pilot testing of a new programme to reveal anticipated and unexpected effects is an important research activity in this phase.

Tool: the programme matrix

The programme matrix aims to facilitate programme development by integrating intervention factors with the behavioural change phases, a strategy adopted by McGuire (1985). The combination of these two results in a programme matrix of 24 cells, each addressing a specific question (De Vries, 1991). Answering all the questions will facilitate the identification of relevant characteristics and issues when developing a programme (Table 6.1). The order of the cells may suggest that one should start with cell 1 and continue from there. However, since many goals of health education programmes are behavioural goals, one often starts by answering the question for cell 21, followed by cells 22–24. The next questions will be those regarding the cognitive changes (cells 9–20), followed by those about the reception and comprehension of information (cells 1–8). The completion of the matrix is an interactive process. For instance, raising the question: 'Who could be the best source to attract attention?' (cell 4) can (further) trigger awareness of important target group characteristics. Application of the matrix also facilitates the analysis of existing programmes.

Testing

The third step is to test the programme's effectiveness. Four types of evaluation questions can be identified. Implementation evaluation describes whether the programme was implemented as intended. Programme evaluation describes the reactions of the target group and programme providers to the programme. Effect evaluation describes the effects of the programme on outcome parameters, such as knowledge, attitudes, encountered social support, self-efficacy, intentions and behaviour. Cost effectiveness describes the relation of the magnitude of the effect and

Table 6.1　The programme matrix for programme evaluation (De Vries, 1991)

Phase	Target group	Message	Channel	Source
Attention	**question 1**: did the target group pay attention to the programme?	**question 2**: did the message stimulate attention to the programme?	**question 3**: did the channels attract attention to the programme?	**question 4**: did the sources stimulate attention to the programme?
Comprehension	**question 5**: did the target group understand the programme and evaluate it positively?	**question 6**: were the messages clear and understandable?	**question 7**: did the channels stimulate comprehension of the programme?	**question 8**: did the sources stimulate comprehension of the programme?
Attitude	**question 9**: did the target group obtain a more positive attitude towards the healthy behaviour?	**question 10**: did the messages discuss the consequences of the healthy and unhealthy behaviours?	**question 11**: were the channels good for discussing the consequences of the healthy and unhealthy behaviour?	**question 12**: were the sources good for discussing the consequences of the healthy and unhealthy behaviour?
Social influences	**question 13**: did the target group obtain (more perceptions of) social support?	**question 14**: did the messages discuss the social influence process and how to obtain support and how to cope with pressure?	**question 15**: were the channels good for discussing the social influence process and how to obtain support and how to cope with pressure?	**question 16**: were the sources good for discussing the social influence process and how to obtain support and how to cope with pressure?
Self-efficacy	**question 17**: did the target group obtain higher levels of self-efficacy?	**question 18**: did the messages discuss how to perform the behaviour and how to cope with the barriers?	**question 19**: were the channels good for discussing how to perform the behaviour and cope with the barriers?	**question 20**: were the sources good for discussing how to perform the behaviour and cope with the barriers?
Behaviour	**question 21**: did the target group adopt the healthy behaviour?	**question 22**: did the programme teach behavioural skills to facilitate the performance of the healthy behaviour?	**question 23**: were the channels good for learning behavioural skills to facilitate performance of the healthy behaviour?	**question 24**: were the sources good for discussing and teaching behavioural skills to facilitate performance of the healthy behaviour?

the costs that were made to realize these effects. Although this step implies some effort and time, it may prevent the dissemination of programmes that are not effective or not cost effective.

The preferred design is a randomized control trial with at least one pretest, random assignment of the groups to the experimental (treatment) and control condition and at least one (but preferably more) post-test. An alternative is a quasi-experimental design where no random assignment of groups to the treatment and control conditions has occurred. By using specific statistical techniques to control for differences between the experimental and control group, these designs can also be used to test health promotion interventions.

In order to understand why a programme did or did not result in the expected changes it is essential to perform process evaluations (Green and Kreuter, 1991; Tones and Tilford, 1994). In process evaluations, the objects of interest are all the programme inputs, the implementation activities and the reactions of stakeholders (Green and Kreuter, 1991). Both quantitative and qualitative techniques are recommended to perform these analyses (Steckler et al., 1992; De Vries et al., 1992).

Continuation

Prevention programmes can only have a significant impact if they are used on a large scale over a substantial period of time. However, development of effective programmes does not automatically imply usage of them on a large scale. The chances of continued utilization can be increased by establishing intersectoral collaboration and support, by developing diffusion strategies and supportive policies.

Intersectoral collaboration

Non-adoption of programmes may be the result of not including relevant stakeholders. Consequently, their ideas may not be represented and they may feel no commitment and ownership. The so-called linkage approach, which is also used in community approaches, may be one way of facilitating their involvement (Havelock, 1971; Bracht, 1990; Orlandi et al., 1990; Dijkstra et al., 1993). However, there is an elaborated variation of this strategy (Figure 6.2).

First, different groups of stakeholders need to be identified and represented in a project group to be able to participate in the process of programme preparation, testing and diffusion. This group consists of (representatives of) persons who have distinct functions:

1. a research group to be responsible for conducting formative and summative evaluations;

2. a resource group to be responsible for providing and developing programme materials;
3. an intermediary group representing programme providers;
4. the target group;
5. a support group consisting of persons who might be able to provide support for the project in one way or another (e.g. youth workers or members of regional councils to help to put the issue on the agenda);
6. a finance group with representatives of those financing the project, to monitor the programme so that it does not conflict with their overall mission.

Second, the motives for participating in the project group need to be analysed in order to be sure that every stakeholder is aware of the advantages of participation. If needed, potential misperceptions need to be corrected and advantages may need further illumination. A precondition for participation is that stakeholders understand what the advantages are (i.e. there have to be certain gains for them).

Third, a consensus should be reached about the level of involvement of each stakeholder in the process of planning, development and implementation of the programme as well as about stakeholders' responsibilities. Finally, it is important to monitor the process of collaboration to verify whether each stakeholder remains satisfied and motivated to participate.

Tool: the linkage matrix

The first step in the linkage approach is to identify relevant stakeholders. The second step is to identify their possible motives for and barriers to collaboration. The steps to apply this approach are listed in Table 6.2.

Diffusion strategies

The first goal of this phase is to study the stimulating and hindering factors (motivational, financial, structural) of programme providers and users regarding the adoption, implementation and continuation of the programme. Therefore, it is important to assess programme providers' evaluations of the programme (Do they understand the advantages of the programme? Do they think that the programme is difficult to use? etc.), as well as their intention to use or not to use the programme. Identifying the facilitating and hindering factors for use enables a diffusion strategy or marketing strategy to 'sell' the programme. This is the second step and therefore refers to programme diffusion.

Supportive strategies

The efficacy of programmes on a larger scale as well as the chances for use can be (partly) dependent on whether the intervention is sufficiently

Table 6.2 The collaboration matrix

	Research group	Resource group	Providers' group	Target group	Support group	Finance group
Who						
Pros of collaboration						
Cons of collaboration						
Support in favour						
Pressure against						
Barriers						

embedded within other existing strategies. Sometimes, the effectiveness of interventions can be neutralized by other competing programmes or policies. For instance, the effects of smoking prevention programmes are diminished and potentially neutralized by national policies that favour smoking (e.g. by allowing tobacco advertisements). This neutralizing effect may also create a negative attitude towards the utilization of such programmes among, for instance, teachers and thus further lower the chances of national adoption. The ultimate effectiveness of programmes therefore cannot be judged in a vacuum and is dependent on other strategies. The continuation of preventive activities may thus be hindered by the fact that necessary conditions, for instance the adoption of school education programmes, may need the support of laws making health education mandatory in schools. Hospitals may need supportive policies to be able to deliver patient education programmes. Similarly, particular health-promoting policies may need the support of information campaigns to educate the population about the need for complying with a particular law. For instance, compliance with safety regulations at work may need additional health education strategies to provide further information about its advantages. In sum, supportive policies may be needed to increase the chances of the adoption of programmes at national levels.

Planning: a circular process

A traditional planning perspective often implies that the problem will be analysed and this will be followed by programme development and implementation. However, the need for stakeholder involvement has already been outlined. Consequently, the creation of a linkage group may have to be the first step in the planning process. Furthermore, the application of the planning model also implies that one may need to go back to some phases in order to reformulate earlier decisions. For instance, the choice of a particular target group may have an impact on the ultimate definition of the problem. The implication is that the planning process can be conceptualized as a circular process with different starting points and that the completion of steps may also influence other steps (Figure 6.1).

THEORIES OF MOTIVATION AND BEHAVIOUR

An important concept in health promotion is motivation and an important assumption is that human beings can be motivated to adopt healthy behaviours. Various theoretical models have been used in health education to understand why human beings undertake specific risk and health behaviours. These will be briefly summarized below.

Social Learning Theory (Bandura, 1986) argues that human behaviour

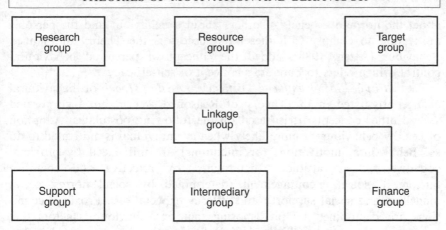

Figure 6.2 The linkage approach.

is the result of an interaction between environmental factors, personal factors and behavioural factors. This interaction is called reciprocal determinism. Environmental factors pertain to the factors that are physically external to a person, such as reinforcements of behaviours by others. The personal factors refer to the abilities of a person to learn from behaviour through their own experiences or through observation of others' behaviour ('vicarious learning') and to several important cognitive variables: self-efficacy expectations, outcome expectations (expectations regarding the consequences of a particular behaviour) and goals or intentions. The behavioural factor refers to the capacities a person has to actually perform a behaviour (i.e. skills, intellectual abilities).

The *Health Belief Model* (Janz and Becker, 1984) was developed in the 1960s and has been elaborated since then. Healthy behaviours are determined by perceived threat, outcome expectations and barriers and cues to action. The perceived threat is a function of a person's perception of the seriousness of the disease and their perceived susceptibility to this disease. The outcomes and barriers refer to the advantages and disadvantages of a particular healthy behaviour. The cues to action activate the awareness of a person about a particular disease and their perception of the threat. In 1988, the concept of self-efficacy was added to the theory.

The *Theory of Reasoned Action* (Fishbein and Ajzen, 1975; Ajzen and Fishbein, 1980) proposes that a person's behaviour can be explained by their intention, provided that the behaviour is under volitional control. The intention is determined by a person's attitude towards this behaviour and a person's social norms. The attitude is determined by a person's beliefs about the consequences of the behaviour and their evaluations of their consequences. The social norm is determined by a person's beliefs about the normative beliefs of others about a behaviour and the person's motivation to comply with these. Its successor, the Theory of Planned Behaviour (Ajzen, 1988), added the concept of perceived behavioural control, which refers to Bandura's concept of self-efficacy.

The *Attitude–Social influence–Efficacy (ASE) Model* of behavioural change originated in the Theory of Reasoned Action but incorporated several other concepts. It is based on the following postulates. Adoption of healthy behaviours is more likely when an individual is motivated to do so. Behavioural motivations (or intentions) are influenced by proximal cognitive factors: attitudes (determined by affective and cognitive outcomes); social encouragement (determined by social norms, social modelling and social support); and efficacy expectations. Proximal cognitions are determined by predisposing factors: behavioural factors (i.e. previous behaviours, skills); biological factors (i.e. gender, age, heredity factors); personality factors (i.e. stress levels, personality factors); social and cultural factors (e.g. socio-economical status, national norms, health-promoting interventions); and physical factors (i.e. a country's climate). Both predisposing factors (e.g. when a behaviour has become routinized) and information can prompt an individual to immediate action, without necessarily influencing the individual's cognitions (De Vries and Kok, 1986; De Vries and Mudde, 1997).

The *Transtheoretical Model* (TTM) shows how the process of behavioural change can be divided into several stages (Prochaska and DiClemente, 1983; Prochaska *et al.*, 1994). People move from precontemplation via contemplation and preparation to action and then to maintenance or relapse. The model has been developed out of research about smoking cessation. The theory describes the importance of two other concepts to understand stage progression: the decisional balance and temptations. The decisional balance refers to the fact that people weigh up the advantages and disadvantages of a particular behaviour (called the 'pros' and 'cons' in TTM). Temptation measures the degree to which people are tempted to revert back to their unhealthy behaviours and this construct is complemented with a self-efficacy scale – both scales refer to a person's level of self-efficacy. A third aspect of TTM is the distinction between cognitive and behavioural processes that influences a person's motivation to change. However, more research about the impact of these processes is needed.

CONCLUSION

The application of a planning model will avoid various pitfalls, such as the development of interventions addressing the wrong determinants, the utilization of materials that are not acceptable for the target group, not working in project groups, not thinking about the consequences for facilitating later national adoption, etc. In the process of health promotion, planning schedules are important to facilitate the successful translation of theory into practice.

REFERENCES

Ajzen, I. (1988) *Attitudes, Personality and Behavior*, Milton Keynes: Open University Press.

Ajzen, I. and Fishbein, M. (1980) *Understanding Attitudes and Predicting Social Behavior*, Englewood Cliffs: Prentice-Hall.

Bandura, A. (1986) *Social Foundations of Thought and Action: a Social Cognitive Theory*, New York: Prentice-Hall.

Bracht, N. (1990) *Health Promotion at the Community Level*, Newbury Park: Sage.

Bracht, N. and Kingsbury, L. (1990) Community organization principles in health promotion: a five-stage model. In N. Bracht, (ed.) *Health Promotion at the Community Level*, Newbury Park: Sage.

De Vries, H. (1989) Towards primary cancer prevention: the Dutch ABC framework. *European Journal for Cancer and Clinical Oncology*, **25**, 1025.

De Vries, H. (1991) *ABCs of Health Education and Promotion; a Manual for the Summer University Course Health Education and Promotion*, Maastricht: Department of Health Education, University of Maastricht.

De Vries, H. and Kok, G.J. (1986) From determinants of smoking behaviour to the implications for a prevention programme. *Health Education Research*, **1**, 85–94.

De Vries, H. and Mudde, A. (1998) Predicting stage transitions for smoking cessation applying the Attitude-Social influence-Efficacy Model. *Psychology and Health* (in press).

De Vries, H., Dijkstra, M. and Kuhlman, P. (1988) Self-efficacy: the third factor besides attitude and subjective norm as a predictor of behavioral intentions. *Health Education Research*, **3**, 273–282.

De Vries, H., Weyts, W., Dijkstra, M. and Kok, G.J. (1992) The utilization of qualitative and quantitative data for health education program planning, implementation and evaluation: a spiral approach. *Health Education Quarterly*, **19**, 101–115.

Dijkstra, M., De Vries, H. and Parcel, G. (1993) The linkage approach applied to a school-based smoking prevention program in the Netherlands. *Journal of School Health*, **63**, 339–342.

Elder, J.P., Geller, E.S., Hovell, M. and Mayer, J.A. (1994) *Motivating Health Behavior*, New York: Delmar.

Fishbein, M. and Ajzen, I. (1975) *Belief, Attitude, Intention and Behavior: an Introduction to Theory and Research*, Reading, MA: Addison-Wesley.

Green, L.W. and Kreuter, M.W. (1991) *Health Promotion Planning; an Educational and Environmental Approach*, Palo Alto, CA: Mayfield.

Green, L.W., Kreuter, M.W., Deeds, S.G. and Partridge, K.B. (1980) *Health Education Planning; a Diagnostic Approach*, Palo Alto, CA: Mayfield.

Havelock, R. (1971) *Planning for Innovation through Dissemination and Utilization of Knowledge*, Ann Arbor: Institute for Social Research.

Janz, N.K. and Becker, M.H. (1984) The Health Belief Model: a decade later. *Health Education Quarterly*, **11**, 1–47.

Kok, G.J. and De Vries, H. (1989) Primary prevention of cancers: the need for health education and intersectoral health promotion. In T. Heller, B. Davey and L. Bailey (eds) *Reducing the Risks of Cancer*, London: Hodder and Stoughton.

Kok, G.J. and Green. L.W. (1990) Research to support health promotion in practice; a plea for increased cooperation. *Health Promotion International*, **5**, 303–308.

Kreuter, M. (1992) PATCH: its origin, basic concepts, and links to contemporary public health policy. *Journal of Health Education*, **23**, 135–139.

McGuire, W.J. (1985) Attitudes and attitude change. In G. Lindzey and E. Aronson (eds) *Handbook of Social Psychology, Vol. II*, New York: Lawrence Erlbaum Associates.

Orlandi, M.A., Landers, C., Weston, R. and Haley, N. (1990) Diffusion of health promotion interventions. In K. Glanz, F.M. Lewis and B.K. Rimer (eds) *Health Behavior and Health Education: Theory, Research and Practice*, San Francisco: Jossey-Bass.

Prochaska, J.O. and DiClemente, C.C. (1983) Stages and processes of self-change of smoking: toward an integrative model of change. *Journal of Consulting and Clinical Psychology*, **51**, 390–395.

Prochaska, J.O., Norcross, J.C. and DiClemente, C.C. (1994) *Changing for Good*, New York: William Morrow.

Rogers, E.M. (1995) *Diffusion of Innovations*, New York: The Free Press.

Sanderson, C., Haglund, B.J., Tillgren, P. *et al.* (1996) Effect and stage models in community intervention programmes and the development of the model for management of intervention programme preparation (MMIPP). *Health Promotion International*, **11**, 143–156.

Steckler, A., McLeroy, K.R., Goodman, R.M., Bird, S.T. and McCormick, L. (1992) Toward integrating qualitative and quantitative methods: an introduction. *Health Education Quarterly*, **19**, 1–8.

Tones, K. and Tilford, S. (1994) *Health Education: Effectiveness, Efficacy and Equity*, 2nd edition, London: Chapman and Hall.

Best practice in cancer control programme evaluation

Afaf Girgis

Cancer control programmes can be delivered via a range of access points, including schools, work places, health care providers, the media and through the whole community and may aim to affect cancer control by encouraging desired outcomes at a number of different levels. Theoretical models of behaviour change may be helpful in designing interventions which are most likely to be effective. For example, the Health Belief Model stipulates that an individual's preparedness to adopt a positive health behaviour is related to the person's perceived severity of the related disease, their perception of personal susceptibility to the disease and the perceived trade-off of costs and benefits associated with adopting the desired behaviour (Rosenstock, 1966, 1974). Therefore, cancer control programmes may attempt to intervene to alter one of these components. For example, smoking control programmes to reduce the rates of smoking by adolescents may intervene at the individual level to improve knowledge and attitudes about smoking (knowledge of severity and susceptibility); at the structural level by enforcing legislation banning tobacco sales to minors (access); or at a more 'macro' level through legislative change increasing the age for the legal purchase of cigarettes (access).

The evaluation strategies used to determine the efficacy and effectiveness of programmes will differ depending on the type of programme, the mode of delivery (access point) and the aims of the evaluation. This chapter will describe some of the evaluation methodologies which are appropriate and present two case studies of different strategies, discussing their advantages and disadvantages.

WHAT TYPE OF EVALUATION IS APPROPRIATE?

Different types of evaluations of cancer control programmes may be undertaken at different stages of programme development and implementation, including process, impact, outcome and economic evaluations. In comprehensive evaluations, a combination of these strategies may be best.

Process evaluation

Process evaluation is usually undertaken if the aims are to determine the degree to which the programme (and/or its individual components) is reaching the target group; participants are satisfied with the programme; all of the components or activities of the programme are being implemented as recommended; and/or the materials and components of the programme are of good quality (Hawe et al., 1990). It is recommended that comprehensive process evaluation be undertaken for all new programmes and for those which have either been substantially modified or are being delivered to a different target group or in a different setting from when they were initially developed.

Process evaluation is particularly important to undertake in conjunction with impact or outcome evaluation, as it helps to explain better both positive and negative intervention effects. For example, if the outcome evaluation (see below) indicates a significant intervention effect, process evaluation may shed light on the components of the intervention programme which contributed to that effect. If outcome evaluations suggest no significant effect, process measures may reveal that the intervention was in fact not fully implemented or that the target group was not adequately reached for the intervention to have impacted optimally. Such information is important in deciding whether to revise the programme (or components of it), rethink how best to deliver it or develop a completely new programme.

Impact and outcome evaluations

The immediate and longer term effects of the programme can be evaluated by undertaking impact and outcome evaluations. The impact of the intervention programme refers to the immediate effects, whilst the outcome refers to longer term effects (Hawe et al., 1990). For example, a comprehensive evaluation of an intervention to reduce skin cancer would measure the short-term effects (impact) of the intervention by assessing changes in the knowledge, attitudes and sun protection practices of community members and the long-term effects (outcome) by assessing changes in the incidence of skin cancer or the deaths from skin cancer as an even longer term outcome. Since changes in incidence and death rates due to cancer control programmes are unlikely to be detected for very long periods of time, the majority of evaluations of cancer control initiatives utilize more immediate or short-term outcomes to determine their efficacy or effectiveness.

Economic evaluations

Given competing priorities in cancer control and potentially limited funds, it is important that economic evaluations are undertaken to determine whether some programmes provide better 'value for money' than others. Such an appraisal compares the resources consumed by a programme (the costs) with the health improvement (the consequences). There are three main types of economic analysis, which are reviewed elsewhere (Torrance, 1986). Briefly, *cost-effectiveness analysis* determines the relationship between observed outcomes and programme costs, expressed as cost per unit of impact achieved (e.g. dollars/pounds per case of disease prevented, dollars/pounds per life year saved, dollars/pounds per life year gained). *Cost-benefit analysis* determines the net social benefit of the programme; and *cost-utility analysis* is a form of cost-effectiveness analysis in which the measure of effect is quality-adjusted life years gained (Torrance, 1986). The type of economic assessment which is most appropriate will depend on the aims of the evaluation and the advice of a health economist should be sought.

WHICH EVALUATION DESIGN IS BEST?

Having decided the primary reasons for the evaluation and identified the most appropriate type to undertake, the next important step is selecting a study design which will adequately meet your aims. Evaluation designs fall into three main categories: non-experimental, quasi-experimental and experimental. These design types have been described in detail in previous publications (Windsor *et al.*, 1984) and have been addressed in previous chapters. The main differences relate to the degree to which the investigator incorporates control strategies (e.g. random allocation to conditions, having a control group) to ensure that intervention effects are in fact due to the intervention rather than to possible confounding or other effects.

Choosing an appropriate evaluation design will depend on its aims and on the importance of having an externally valid outcome, i.e. an outcome which can be generalized to groups other than those in your study. For example, if you are trialling a programme on a small scale (e.g. a schools programme in one region) with the hope of introducing it on a larger scale (e.g. state-wide) if it is effective, then external validity is important. In the following section, two case studies are presented to highlight the relative merits of different evaluation designs. These should provide a useful guide to choosing an appropriate design for evaluating your programme.

When cancer control programmes are developed, one of the important evaluation components is to assess the acceptability of the intervention to the target group and the strategy for delivering this intervention. The first case study describes such an evaluation. A more complex type of evaluation design is described in case study 2, a controlled trial to evaluate the efficacy and cost effectiveness of a community-wide cancer control programme, using a matched pairs design.

CASE STUDY 1: UTILIZATION AND ACCEPTABILITY OF WRITTEN HEALTH EDUCATION MATERIALS

(*Source*: Newell, S., Girgis, A. and Sanson-Fisher, R.W. (1995) Recall, retention, utilization and perceived acceptability of written health education materials. *Australian Journal of Public Health*, **19**(4), 368–374.)

Background and objectives

This publication describes an evaluation of the impact of two distribution strategies on the recall of receipt of health education materials (on cancer and cardiovascular disease) and the retention, utilization and perceived acceptability of the materials. The two strategies examined were mailout and personal distribution by health care professionals, which the researchers selected based on evidence that they appear to be the most commonly used strategies. The paper provides a good rationale for undertaking this kind of assessment: written health education materials are a frequently used intervention tool in the field of health promotion and disease prevention and how they are received could affect the way in which they are perceived by recipients. It appears that, whilst much research has been conducted to produce concrete and specific guidelines about how to design such materials in order to make them easy and interesting to read and credible to the reader, the issue of the impact of the method of distribution on how well such materials are received has been less well studied. Furthermore, the costs of these strategies may be quite different. Hence, the researchers also attempted to estimate the cost effectiveness of the two strategies in order to determine which provided better value for money.

This formative evaluation was undertaken as a pilot study to determine the best distribution method to use for a larger controlled trial of the evaluation of the health education materials. Such evaluations are very important and are recommended for cancer control programmes where there may be a number of possible delivery strategies or where the efficacy of the chosen delivery strategy in reaching the target group has not yet been demonstrated.

Intervention

To test the two distribution strategies, 300 people received the education materials through the mail in a personally addressed envelope; another 212 received the materials from their general practitioner at the end of a routine consultation. All participants received exactly the same package of materials containing:

1. an introductory letter which explained the need for people to adopt preventive behaviours and engage in screening behaviours that would reduce their risk of developing cancer and cardiovascular disease;
2. a 'Better Health Booklet' – a 16-page booklet which provided information about the prevalence of cancer and cardiovascular disease; recommendations about preventive, screening and early detection behaviours and details about where to go for further information. The readability of the booklet was assessed and more than 86% of adults resident in the study region met this educational requirement (CDATA, 1991);
3. a 'Better Health Diary' – a purse/wallet-sized diary with space for recording health information (such as blood group and family history of cancer and cardiovascular disease) and an individual's screening history.

Evaluation design

The evaluation design was a simple descriptive study. Structured interviews were conducted once with randomly selected individuals two weeks after they had received the materials. To reduce the chances of contamination between the mailout and the general practitioner groups, two geographically discrete, semi-rural communities in New South Wales (NSW), Australia, were selected for participation in the study. These communities were selected on the basis of their proximity to the research group and provided a relatively small and localized sample. This would, in other circumstances, be a potential source of selection bias which could limit the generalizability of the results to the general population. However, the communities in this study were chosen to provide information about small, rural communities for a larger controlled trial and, therefore, the generalizability of the outcomes to other target groups was not important.

In this trial, use of a control group was not important as the aim of this pilot study was to compare the effects of two distribution strategies with each other, rather than to quantify the effect *per se*. Case study 2 presents a trial where the incorporation of a control group was vital to the aims of the evaluation.

Data collection instruments

McGuire's Communication Persuasion Model was used as a framework for assessing the response to the materials (McGuire, 1984). This model describes a series of steps whereby individuals change their behaviour in response to an educational message: exposure to the message, attention to the message, interest in the message, comprehension of the message, skill acquisition, yielding to the message, retention and retrieval of the message and, finally, behaviour change. Furthermore, the survey employed in this study was closely based on a survey used previously by the research team and found to be acceptable for evaluating the effectiveness of written health education materials (Paul, 1994).

The range of issues covered in the survey adequately addressed the aims of the evaluation. It assessed participants' recall of receipt of the materials; their reported retention of the booklet and diary; reported utilization of the booklet (how much of the booklet they had read and which sections were found to be the most and least useful); and reported utilization of the diary (which sections of the diary they had completed). The perceived acceptability of the materials to participants was also assessed to allow for modification, if warranted, prior to the main study. In addition to the measures of acceptability and use of the materials, the researchers assessed participants' knowledge and attitudes regarding issues in the booklet. A rationale is provided for collecting this information, since the items may be potential predictors of utilization according to the Health Belief Model of behaviour change (Rosenstock, 1966, 1974). Information about participants' demographic characteristics was also collected as potential predictors of the outcomes of interest.

One potential source of response bias in this evaluation was the use of self-report to assess respondents' retention and utilization of the materials. Whilst self-report is of unknown accuracy, the researchers used a number of safeguards, including asking respondents who reported having read any of the booklet which sections they considered to be the most useful and asking those who reported having written in their diaries to bring them to the phone and tell the interviewer which sections they had completed. In both cases, the results suggest that inaccurate reporting was not a major problem in this study. In addition, should such inaccuracies exist, there was no reason to expect differential rates of inaccuracies from the two groups. Therefore, whilst such a bias may affect the generalizability of the results to other groups, it is not a problem in terms of the aims of this evaluation. In case study 2, where one of the aims is to collect prevalence data, response bias would present a significant problem as it would limit the ability to generalize the results or to compare the prevalence data with other groups.

Study samples

In the GP group, 212 consecutive patients who met the researchers' eligibility criteria were approached for consent to be contacted by phone to participate in a survey. Of these, 165 were contactable during the period of the study and consented to complete the telephone survey, giving an overall consent rate of 82.9% from the patients approached and contactable during the study period. In the mailout group, the names of 300 people (150 males, 150 females) aged 20–60 years were randomly selected from the electoral register and all were sent the materials. Of these, 258 (86%) were still at the same address and contactable during the study period and 221 (85.7%) of these consented to complete the telephone survey. These represent relatively high participation rates, minimizing the potential for selection bias from this source.

However, one potential source of bias is that individuals were not randomly allocated to the experimental conditions: rather, one community was assigned to GP distribution and the other to mailout distribution, raising the question of clustering. In other words, it is possible that individuals in each community would have reacted differently to the materials irrespective of the distribution method involved. While the researchers acknowledge this as a possibility, they have provided various reasons for believing that this would be unlikely to account for the large differences found between the groups. However, this is an important issue to consider when planning an evaluation design. A decision needs to be made by individual evaluators regarding the importance of having outcomes with external validity. Case study 2 presents an alternative design which takes the possibility of clustering into consideration.

A second possible source of sampling bias is that this study compared two slightly different samples: one was a general population sample and the other was a patient sample. This is not believed to be a significant problem in this study as approximately 80% of the NSW population see a medical practitioner at least once every 12 months (Australian Bureau of Statistics, 1992), a proportion not dissimilar to the 86% of the population eligible for inclusion in the electoral register (CDATA, 1991). Evaluators should, however, be aware of the potential bias introduced by comparing different samples.

Statistical tests

Chi square analyses were conducted to assess whether any demographic differences existed between respondents in the two groups; whether any significant differences existed in the recall, retention, utilization and perceived acceptability rates between respondents in the two groups; and whether a number of variables were associated with booklet utilization across the two groups. These are appropriate analyses for these types of data. Furthermore, the size of the samples in this study will allow a difference of 15% or greater to be detected between conditions.

Studies such as this one, where a large number of statistical analyses are being performed, are at risk of a type I error. Such an error would result in rejecting the null hypothesis (i.e. no difference) when, in fact, the null hypothesis is true (Pagano and Gauvreau, 1993). As a number of hypotheses were being tested in this study, the researchers adjusted the critical p value to minimize the likelihood of a type I error.

Basic cost-effectiveness ratios can be calculated relatively easily and should be considered as a useful addition to evaluation designs which involve comparisons of at least two strategies or interventions. In this study, the costs of designing the materials were excluded from the cost-effectiveness analyses as these are fixed costs and would not be affected by distribution method or the number of booklets produced. For the mailout group, the total cost of printing, packaging, mailout preparation and postage was estimated and for the general practitioner group, the total cost of printing, packaging and delivering the booklets to the general practitioners was estimated. A cost-effectiveness ratio was then calculated per booklet read for the two strategies. While more complex cost-effectiveness analyses can be undertaken, this simple analysis was sufficient to address the evaluation aims of this study. Case study 2 describes more complex cost analyses, which were warranted for the aims of that evaluation.

Conclusions

The analyses undertaken led the researchers to conclude that general practitioner distribution led to higher rates of receipt and retention of the materials. However, mailout distribution, via the electoral register, led to higher utilization rates and allowed access to a larger proportion of the population, resulting in more individuals having been exposed to the education message. The evaluation design, sampling frame and statistical analyses used in this study are appropriate and give no cause to reject the researchers' conclusions.

Summary

- The development of the intervention materials was based on theoretical models of behaviour change. Furthermore, preliminary evaluation of the materials, including readability levels, was undertaken to ensure their appropriateness for the target group.
- Contamination between intervention conditions was minimized by using two discrete communities.
- The sample selection may potentially be a source of bias, although in

this case, the researchers have provided arguments to suggest this was not a significant problem.

- The researchers acknowledged the possibility of a type 1 error due to the large number of analyses and adjusted the *p* value to reduce this likelihood.
- The inclusion of an economic appraisal provides important information and is simple enough to incorporate into these types of evaluations.
- This study design was appropriate for the type of formative evaluation described in this publication.

CASE STUDY 2: EFFICACY AND COST EFFECTIVENESS OF A COMMUNITY ACTION PROGRAMME

(*Source*: Hancock, L., Sanson-Fisher, R., Redman, S. *et al.* (1996) Community action for cancer prevention: overview of the Cancer Action in Rural Towns (CART) project. *Health Promotion International,* **11**(4), 277–290.

Background and objectives

This publication describes the rationale, aims, design and methods of a community action project, Cancer Action in Rural Towns **(CART)**, which attempts to meet the methodological specifications necessary to evaluate effectively this approach to encouraging health behaviour change. The paper focuses on the evaluation of the CART project, which was under way at the time of publication.

The primary aim of the CART project is to explore the effectiveness of a community action programme in increasing community rates of preventive and screening behaviours relating to breast, cervical, smoking-related and skin cancer in rural towns in one Australian state. The specific aims are:

1. to describe current rates of preventive and screening behaviours for breast, cervical, smoking-related and skin cancers in rural communities in the state of New South Wales (NSW), Australia;
2. to explore the effectiveness of a community action programme in increasing community rates of preventive and screening behaviours relating to breast, cervical, smoking-related and skin cancers when compared with control rural communities;
3. to monitor the economic and financial costs of community action programmes for individuals and service providers;
4. to undertake an economic appraisal in order to assess the cost effec-

tiveness of a community action programme in comparison to other strategies;

5. to describe the implementation of the community action programme and to assess its acceptability to participating communities;
6. to develop a strategy and resource materials which could be used to implement community action programmes relating to cancer in other rural communities.

Intervention

The CART project involved a community-wide intervention delivered via a range of access points (schools, work places, community organizations, health care providers, retailers and media). It involved the formation of community committees and the utilization of access-point networks to initiate and maintain intervention strategies within each intervention town, an approach which was reportedly developed with reference to past similar projects (Puska, 1984; COMMIT Research Group, 1991; Knight et al., 1994) and through consultation with identified experts in the field, local health promotion workers and lay people.

This type of intervention is necessarily complex as not all communities would be expected to adopt the intervention uniformly. To minimize possible differences, the research team approach to towns was standardized and materials for activating the intervention were provided by the research team to encourage similar activities in each experimental town. A community facilitator (NSW Cancer Council Health Education Officers with experience in community-based cancer reduction strategies) was recruited for each intervention town, with the main role of acting as a link between the community and the research team. CART was then introduced to each intervention town through an open invitation community meeting, at which a Community Committee was formed. The CART Committee was asked at the first meeting to nominate representatives to take responsibility for activation through six key access points: health care providers, community organizations, media, retailers, schools and work places. These access-point networks were the main vehicle of the CART intervention and the research team intended that as many people from the community as possible be involved in the intervention at this level. To assist these groups, standard strategy packages were developed which outlined recommendations for activities in each access point based on the likelihood of their efficacy. Resource packages with pamphlets, posters, draft letters and other resources were provided for each access point, to aid in conducting activities.

Given the nature of the intervention, it was expected that activities and time frames would vary considerably between towns. Therefore, the researchers undertook careful monitoring of intervention activity in each town to allow a detailed description of the intervention to be given and also to allow for variations in the intervention process to be used as potential confounders in the evaluation analysis. Process measures for the project included media monitoring, measures of change in institutional policies, records of CART intervention activities and details on non-intervention activities within experimental and control towns.

Although the flexibility in the components and time frames of the intervention in participating towns was seen as a key to securing and maintaining community involvement, the differential effects of components of the intervention undertaken in the different towns are difficult to quantify. Therefore, the results of the evaluation will indicate whether a community action approach is effective in increasing cancer control but will not identify components of such an approach which may be more effective than others. Whilst such information is important, it was not a specific aim of this study.

For other programmes, where it may be important to know which intervention components worked more effectively, a number of alternative evaluation designs are available. Where resources are available, a randomized controlled trial is the most rigorous strategy, with a control group and a number of experimental groups. In this case, the number of experimental groups would depend on the number of different components the researchers wanted to test. For example, in a trial of the effectiveness of strategies to increase cervical screening, three experimental groups were included in the evaluation to determine the effectiveness of television media alone, versus media combined with a letter of invitation to attend for screening, versus media combined with GP-based recruitment (Byles *et al.*, 1994).

In some cases where an equivalent control condition is difficult to establish or funds for undertaking the evaluation do not permit it, time series analysis can be utilized (Hawe *et al.*, 1990). This basically involves taking lots of measures over a certain time period, which should include sufficient pre-intervention observations to plot the natural changes and the size and direction of these, occurring in the group. Observations throughout and following the introduction of the intervention will allow the researchers to identify effects which differ from the natural pre-intervention observations. Byles *et al.* (1995) provide a good example of this design for evaluating a cervical cancer intervention.

Evaluation design

A difficult methodological issue for community action programmes is the establishment of adequate control groups, because whole communities rather than individuals must be assigned to control and treatment groups (cluster randomization) and many communities must be assigned to each group (Donner, 1987; Donner *et al.*, 1987). As acknowledged by the authors, evaluation designs which involve only one or two treatment communities cannot exclude the possibility that changes in behaviour are due to factors other than the intervention (Koepsell *et al.*, 1991).

To overcome this, the CART project adopted a matched pairs design, with pre- and post- outcome measures. One town from each matched pair (ten pairs) was randomly allocated to either the experimental or control condition. The authors report that the sample of 20 towns (ten matched pairs) was based on feasibility and financial considerations. However, on advice from experts, this was considered to be a sufficient sample to answer the aims of the project, with significant improvements in the direction of the intervention towns needing to be demonstrated in at least eight of the ten pairs for the intervention to be considered successful. The probability of obtaining this result given no baseline difference between towns, is reported to be 5% (Donner, 1987).

The selection of the 20 rural towns for inclusion in the study involved a series of steps to ensure that the pairs of towns were well matched and that contamination between study groups due to proximity of the intervention to control towns was minimized. This is described in detail in the publication. The matching variables, which were selected following extensive consultation with statistical and methodological experts both in Australia and overseas, were demographic structure (including age distribution, ethnicity, occupation, education levels and non-English-speaking background); population density as an isolation index; and average summer temperature.

The process used to ensure that town pairs were well matched was quite thorough and comprehensive, minimizing the possibility of sample selection as a source of bias. However, baseline levels of cancer control behaviours in the communities were not available prior to the start of the intervention period and may not have been similar in the matched town pairs, introducing another source of bias. This study is not dissimilar to many cancer control programme evaluations, where one of the components of the evaluation is to collect baseline data. Hence, this variable is often not available at the time of matching of study groups. However, various statistical methods are available to take into consideration any baseline differences between study groups to ensure that outcomes of the evaluation are valid. A statistician should be consulted in these cases.

Data collection instruments

Given the short time frame for outcome measurement, changes in health outcomes such as cancer incidence would not be expected (Hawe *et al.*, 1990). The effectiveness of the community action programme will be evaluated using a traditional pre–post data collection procedure, comparing

Table 7.1 Summary of outcome targets and evaluation measures for the CART project

Cancer	Outcome To examine if the community action programme results in:	Measure	Sample size per town
Breast	An increase in the number of women (50–69 years) receiving screening mammograms	Adult Cohort Study (self-report)	$n = 1000$
Cervical	An increase in the number of women (not screened in the previous 2 years) receiving cervical cancer screening (Pap tests)	Health Insurance Commission Pap test rates (objective)	Three-monthly statistics for five years pre-intervention and throughout the intervention period
Smoking-related	A decrease in the number of adolescents who begin to smoke	Cross-sectional school-based self-report survey, with bogus pipeline enhancement	$n = 200$ (all years 9 and 10 students from all secondary schools)
	An increase in the proportion of adult smokers who quit	Adult Cohort Study smoker self-report of quitting	$n = 150$ current smokers
Skin: protection	An increase in the proportion of secondary school children who use solar protection	Cross-sectional school-based survey using diary self-report of weekend behaviour (validated measure)	$n = 200$ from each secondary school Whole classes randomly selected
	An increase in the proportion of people who use solar protection at community swimming pools and recreation areas	Direct observation of solar protection behaviours at swimming pools and recreational areas (objective)	$n = 200$
	A decrease in acquisition of pigmented naevi on the backs of primary school children	Photograph naevi counts of backs for 5–7-year-olds (validated measure)	$n = 60$
Skin: detection	An increase in the number of skin biopsies	Health Insurance Commission skin biopsy rates (objective)	Three-monthly statistics for five years pre-intervention and throughout the intervention period

changes in health risk behaviours from baseline to follow-up and between study conditions. Economic analyses are also undertaken.

Changes in the outcomes of interest in relation to cervical, skin, breast and smoking-related cancers were assessed using a number of strategies: self-report measures of adult smoking quit rates, health insurance commission provider presentations data, surveys of adolescent smoking and solar protection practices, and direct observation of solar protection practices at schools and community venues, as summarized in Table 7.1. Many of the measures involved an independent assessment (e.g. direct observations) or utilized validated instruments (e.g. sun protection diary). However, self-report may be a possible source of response bias. To minimize this, the researchers incorporated strategies to enhance self-report where possible, such as the use of a bogus pipeline for the measure of adolescent smoking.

Economic evaluations to determine whether community action represents 'value for money' within the context of the Australian health care system are the subject of subsequent papers. However, the researchers appear to be applying well-founded methods to evaluate different aspects of the CART project: cost-effectiveness analysis (Drummond *et al.*, 1987); travel cost method (Acton, 1975); and contingent valuation method (Johannesson *et al.*, 1991).

Study samples and statistical tests

Sample size calculations for each outcome measure were performed using a formula which takes into account the clustering effect introduced by having whole communities as the unit of interest. Alpha was set at 0.05 and the intra-town correlation coefficient (rho) for each outcome variable was calculated from baseline data (Snedecor and Cochran, 1980; Hsieh, 1988). The sample sizes for each of the measures per town are shown in Table 1. These samples are large enough to allow detection of relatively small differences which may be expected from this type of intervention: as small as 5% in the smoking outcomes and 10% in the sun protection outcomes, given the calculated rho values and a power of 90%. Appropriate analyses are proposed for this sampling design and clustering effects and logistic procedures are employed to explore the predictors of the hypothesized changes.

Potential confounders

If an intervention effect is detected, the relative contribution to this effect of other cancer control programmes (including research or public health initiatives) would be difficult to determine. Such external influences may in fact mask any intervention trends. The researchers have attempted to detail such potential confounders with the proposed process measures, which should identify any additional activities occurring in both the experimental and control towns. Therefore, although unable to control this, the researchers can document it.

Summary

- The town selection and matching procedures were rigorous and aimed to reduce the likelihood of confounding or contamination between study conditions.
- The towns were randomly allocated to the study group, reducing the likelihood of bias.
- The sample sizes (towns and participants within towns) were sufficient to detect statistically and clinically significant changes in the outcomes of interest and the proposed statistical analyses are appropriate to address the aims of the evaluation.
- The intervention was still under way at the time of publication, but the process to date was well described. Furthermore, process measures will facilitate the detailed description of the intervention in each experimental town. It is not clear whether an intervention period of three years would be sufficient to detect important cancer control changes across whole communities.
- The planned process measures were comprehensive and would allow a reasonable description of the intervention in each of the experimental towns, as well as identification of possible confounders such as cancer control initiatives external to the project.
- The majority of the outcome measures used were either objective or had previously been validated.
- The inclusion of an economic appraisal will provide information about the relative cost effectiveness of this approach compared to others. This information is very important in a climate of competing demands on resources for cancer control initiatives.
- This study design was appropriate for evaluating the cancer control strategy described in the publication. However, the generalizability of the results is limited to rural towns of a similar size.

Whilst these case studies only present two examples of evaluation designs, the concepts described (e.g. the need for control groups, valid measures, etc.) should assist evaluators to identify the most appropriate design to suit their purposes. Hawe *et al.* (1990) provide further detail on different evaluation designs.

REFERENCES

Acton, J.P. (1975) Non-monetary factors in the demand for medical services: some empirical evidence. *Journal of Political Economy*, **83**(3), 595.

Australian Bureau of Statistics. (1992) 1989–90 *National Health Survey: Health Related Actions* (catalogue number 4375.0), Canberra: Australian Government Publishing Service.

Byles, J.E., Sanson-Fisher, R.W., Redman, S., Dickinson, J.A. and Halpin, S. (1994) Effectiveness of three community based strategies to promote screening for cervical cancer. *Journal of Medical Screening*, 1, 150–158.

Byles, J.E., Redman, S., Sanson-Fisher, R.W. and Boyle, C.A. (1995) Effectiveness of two direct-mail strategies to encourage women to have cervical (Pap) smears. *Health Promotion International*, 10(1), 5–15.

CDATA (1991) With Supermap (Catalogue Number 2721.0) (computer programme), Canberra: Australian Bureau of Statistics.

COMMIT Research Group. (1991) Community Intervention Trial for Smoking Cessation (COMMIT): summary of design and intervention. *Journal of the National Cancer Institute*, 83(22), 1620.

Donner, A. (1987) Statistical methodology for paired cluster designs. *American Journal of Epidemiology*, 126, 972.

Donner, A., Birkett, N. and Buck, C. (1987) Randomization of cluster: sample size requirements and analysis. *American Journal of Epidemiology*, 114, 906.

Drummond, N.W., Stoddart, G.L. and Torrance, G.W. (1987) *Methods for the Economic Evaluation of Health Care Programmes*, Oxford: Oxford Medical Publications.

Hawe, P., Degeling, D. and Hall, J. (1990) *Evaluating Health Promotion*, Sydney: MacLennan and Petty.

Hsieh, F.H. (1988) Sample size formulas for intervention studies with the cluster as unit of randomization. *Statistics in Medicine*, 7, 1195.

Johannesson, M., Jonsson, B. and Borgquist, L. (1991) Willingness to pay for anti-hypertensive therapy: results of a Swedish pilot study. *Journal of Health Economics*, 10(4), 461.

Knight, J., Bowman, J., Considine, R. *et al.* (1994) The Adolescent Project: reducing adolescent smoking and unsafe drinking in rural towns in the Hunter area of NSW. *Health Promotion Journal*, 4(1), 54.

Koepsell, T.D., Martin, D.C., Diehr, P.H. *et al.* (1991) Data analysis and sample size issues in evaluation of community-based health promotion and disease prevention programs: a mixed-model analysis of variance approach. *Journal of Clinical Epidemiology*, 44(7), 701.

McGuire, W.J. (1984) Public communication as a strategy for inducing health-promoting behavioural change. *Preventive Medicine*, 13, 299–319.

Pagano, M. and Gauvreau, K. (1993) *Principles of Biostatistics*, California: Duxbury Press.

Paul, C.L. (1994) The development of printed health education messages (dissertation). Newcastle, NSW: University of Newcastle.

Puska, P. (1984). Community based prevention of cardiovascular disease: the North Kareia Project. In J.D. Matarazzo (ed.) *A Handbook of Health Enhancement and Disease Prevention*, New York: John Wiley.

Rosenstock, I.M. (1966) Why people use health services. *Milbank Memorial Fund Quarterly*, 44(suppl), 94–127.

Rosenstock, I.M. (1974) The health belief model and preventive behaviour. *Health Education Monographs*, **4**, 27–59.

Snedecor, G.S. and Cochran, W.G. (1980) *Statistical Methods*, Ames: Iowa State University Press.

Torrance, G.W. (1986) *Measurement of Health State Utilities for Economic Appraisal: A Review*, Amsterdam: Elsevier.

Windsor, R.A., Baranowski, T., Clark, N. and Cutter, G. (1984) *Evaluation of Health Promotion and Education Programs*, Palo Alto, CA: Mayfield.

8 Evidence-based health promotion

John Wiggers and Rob Sanson-Fisher

INTRODUCTION

The contribution of research evidence to health promotion has gained increasing attention over the past decade (Flay, 1986; Glanz *et al.*, 1996). Despite this, the role and value of research evidence in informing health promotion practice is the subject of considerable debate (Anonymous, 1996). This debate can be attributed in part to health promotion having its origins in a variety of disciplines (Green and Kreuter, 1991; Downie *et al.*, 1996) and, as a consequence, involving the application of a wide range of philosophies and strategies to improve the health of individuals and populations.

Despite its diversity of history and methodology, health promotion practice is dependent upon evidence as a determinant of its activity. When planning a health promotion initiative, the health promotion practitioner applies anecdotal, research and other forms of evidence when determining the type of initiative to be undertaken. The role of evidence *per se* is therefore not so much the focus of debate as is the nature and quality of evidence used to inform the decision-making process. It is in this context that a systematic application of quality research evidence is suggested to improve the selection of appropriate health promotion initiatives and hence improve the likelihood of the community obtaining a health benefit (Anonymous, 1996).

Several models have been proposed which identify the decision-making questions central to determining the focus of health promotion activity (Nutbeam *et al.*, 1990, Green and Kreuter, 1991; Sanson-Fisher and Campbell, 1994; Winett, 1995; Oldenburg *et al.*, 1996). One of these, the

Staged Approach to Health Promotion (Sanson-Fisher and Campbell, 1994), is described in this chapter as a tool for systematically applying quality research evidence to the planning and conduct of health promotion activities. The application of the model will be described with reference to a commonly accepted goal of health promotion: reducing the prevalence of smoking (Nutbeam *et al.*, 1993; Canadian Taskforce on the Periodic Health Examination, 1994).

Health promotion practice does not necessarily proceed in an ordered fashion. There are occasions where expressed community need for action requires a more rapid response than can be provided by following a series of structured decision-making steps. Nonetheless, in overall terms, a logical decision-making approach incorporating quality research evidence is considered to be more likely to produce a sustained improvement in the health of the community and is therefore more ethically and professionally responsible. In clinical medicine, a new pharmacological treatment is not incorporated into practice without rigorous research establishing its need, benefit, absence of harm and practical feasibility. In principle, new health promotion initiatives should similarly not be implemented without equivalent supporting data.

WHAT IS EVIDENCE-BASED HEALTH PROMOTION?

The planning and conduct of health promotion activities involves a staged decision-making process concerned with: the identification of health-related problems and needs in the community; the selection of interventions intended to redress these problems and needs; the assessment of intervention effectiveness and methods to achieve the widespread adoption of efficacious interventions. Evidence-based health promotion involves the explicit application of quality research evidence when making such decisions. Research evidence may be obtained from appraisal of the research literature or, where feasible, from research data collected by the health promotion practitioner. Evidence-based health promotion involves more than reading, appraising or collecting research data on an *ad hoc* basis, undertaken as a matter of interest or professional development. Rather, it involves the appraisal or collection of research data being systematically integrated into and directed by the health promotion decision-making process.

The application of quality research evidence to planning and conducting health promotion initiatives must occur in conjunction with the application of the health promotion practitioner's professional skills and knowledge. Such professional expertise involves not only the technical capacity to select health issues, target groups, interventions and evaluation designs, but also the ability to identify and respond to the expressed needs and circumstances of communities, governments and interest groups. Evidence-based health promotion therefore comprises a decision-making process whereby quality research evidence is applied in a manner consistent with the circumstances of a community, their expressed need for intervention, the priorities of government and funding authorities and the availability of resources. Neither quality research evidence nor professional expertise alone is a sufficient basis for appropriate and effective health promotion.

WHY IS THERE A NEED FOR EVIDENCE-BASED HEALTH PROMOTION?

A more explicit and systematic incorporation of quality research evidence into the planning and conduct of health promotion initiatives is required for a number of reasons. First, developments in knowledge that arise from research frequently lead to major changes in the direction and content of health promotion practice. For example, the demonstration by Russell *et al.* (1979) of the efficacy of brief intervention techniques for smoking cessation has had a dramatic influence on health promotion initiatives directed not only at smoking cessation, but also at modifying other risk behaviours such as alcohol consumption (Fleming *et al.*, 1997). Lack of awareness of or failure to incorporate such research evidence in health promotion practice reduces the likelihood that the community will obtain the greatest possible benefits from scarce health promotion resources.

Second, health promotion practitioners do not routinely incorporate new health promotion research findings into their practice (Maclean and Eakin, 1992; National Health Strategy, 1993; Redman, 1996; Oldenburg *et al.*, 1996). To date, health promotion practitioners have relied upon tradi-tional methods of continuing professional education as a means of acquir-ing new research knowledge. These methods, including conference attendance and non-systematic reading of texts and journals have been shown to be deficient in keeping health care practitioners up to date (Haynes *et al.*, 1984; Covell *et al.*, 1985; Antman *et al.*, 1992; Davis *et al.*, 1995). As a consequence, the capacity of practitioners to apply current knowledge is constrained, reducing the likelihood of the community obtaining the greatest benefit from existing research effort (Sibley *et al.*, 1982; Evans *et al.*, 1986; Ramsey *et al.*, 1991; Davis *et al.*, 1995). To over-come these limitations, a more systematic approach to incorporating research evidence into the planning and conduct of health promotion initiatives is required.

Finally, the practice of health promotion faces an increasing stringency of resource allocation and an increased demand to demonstrate its capa-city to achieve desired health outcomes. As a consequence, the practice of health promotion has become more focused on those activities that are most likely to produce a health gain for the community. In adopting such a focus, a much greater emphasis is placed on: the selection of measurement strategies demonstrated to be accurate in measuring health status; the identification of population groups with the greatest need; and the identification of intervention strategies demonstrated to be effective.

WHAT IS QUALITY RESEARCH EVIDENCE?

As evidenced-based practice involves a systematic process of applying research evidence to professional decision-making (Rosenberg and Donald, 1995), different forms of evidence are required for different decision-making steps. In the case of seeking to identify the most accurate measure of health risk status, evidence-based practice involves the appraisal or collection of research data from appropriately designed cross-sectional studies that compare the measure of interest to a 'gold-standard' measure (Sackett *et al.*, 1997). When identifying the nature and distribution of health issues in a population, evidence-based health promotion involves the practitioner appraising the findings of both quantitative and qualitative descriptive studies.

When seeking to identify an appropriate form of intervention, evidence-based practice involves the appraisal of studies that minimize the likelihood of biased results. As the results of non-experimental research studies are more likely to be biased and randomized controlled trials less likely to be so, the latter are accepted as the preferred source of information (Last, 1995). However, the conduct of evidence-based health promotion requires a flexible approach as not all forms of intervention require randomized controlled trials and in many instances, such trials cannot be undertaken for ethical and logistic reasons. Similarly, given the relatively recent focus on the role of randomized trials in professional decision making, trial results are not available for many forms of available intervention. In these instances, information is sought from the next best source of evidence.

Hierarchy of evidence for the selection of health promotion interventions

An accepted hierarchy of research evidence quality has been developed for assessing the effectiveness of preventive interventions in primary care settings (Woolf *et al.*, 1990; Last, 1995). Such a hierarchy has subsequently been adapted to provide a basis for assessing the quality of more broadly focused health promotion interventions (NHS Centre for Reviews and Dissemination, 1996), as illustrated in Table 8.1.

In *randomized controlled trials*, participants are allocated randomly to either an experimental group that receives an intervention or a control group that does not. Both groups are followed prospectively to determine

Table 8.1 Hierarchy of research evidence quality (Source: NHS Centre for Reviews and Dissemination, 1996)

Level	Source of research evidence
I	At least one properly designed randomized controlled trial
II-1	Well-designed controlled trials without randomization. Quasi-experimental studies
II-2	Well-designed cohort (prospective) studies, preferably from more than one centre or research group
II-3	Well-designed case-control (retrospective) studies, preferably from more than one centre or research group
III	Large differences in comparisons between times and/or locations, with or without intervention
IV	Opinions of respected authorities, based on clinical experience, descriptive studies, or reports of expert committees

whether changes occur in the outcome of interest. Random allocation of participants is undertaken to ensure the greatest possible similarity between the groups by distributing known and unknown confounding factors randomly and, as hoped for, equally between the groups. In this way, the validity of attributing observed study outcomes to the effects of the intervention can be maximized. The validity of inferences concerning the effect of an intervention can be enhanced by blinding either the participants, the researcher or both to the allocation of participants to groups.

Controlled trials without randomization and quasi-experimental studies are more likely to be biased, primarily due to the non-random allocation of participants to an intervention. As a consequence, the likelihood of systematic differences between those who receive an intervention and those who do not is increased, reducing the validity and generalizability of the results.

In *cohort studies* the allocation of participants to groups that receive or do not receive an intervention is not determined by the researcher. In such studies, individuals who have been exposed to an intervention independent of the research process are followed prospectively and compared with a group of participants who have not been exposed. Given that participants are not allocated randomly to either group, systematic differences between the groups may bias the study outcomes. The effect of such a bias may be limited by controlling for known confounding factors. However, as it is not possible to control for unknown confounding factors in such a design, the validity and generalizability of the results are reduced.

In contrast to the prospective design of controlled trials and cohort studies, *case-control studies* retrospectively assess whether participants who have an identified disease/need differ from those who have not with regard to exposure to a risk or intervention. The validity of any inferences drawn from such studies is reduced by: the inability to control for confounding variables; observer bias as the researcher is aware of the study outcome; recall bias as the participant is required to recall past events; and selection bias as those who have the condition/risk/need may differ systematically from those who do not.

The remaining *uncontrolled* sources of research evidence are considered appropriate for describing differences in disease/risk rates between groups but do not provide strong evidence concerning the effectiveness of an intervention or the effect of an agent or risk factor on health outcome. Such studies may suggest improvements in outcomes coincident with the introduction of an intervention or agent. However, in the absence of controls, such improvements can be equally attributed to secular changes as to the effect of the intervention itself.

Although the above hierarchy provides an overall indication of the relative quality of evidence from intervention-based research, further consideration needs to be applied when interpreting study results. For example, although a randomized controlled trial may suggest a positive health outcome from an intervention, such results may be an artefact of measurement error or inappropriate participant selection, rather than a positive effect of the intervention itself. Similarly, the absence of significant findings may reflect too small a sample size or an inadequate follow-up of participants, rather than an ineffective intervention. Appraisal of the quality of the study therefore remains an important imperative in addition to appraising its design.

Systematic reviews

Not all health promotion practitioners have the time, the resources or the skills to routinely appraise the research literature when undertaking health promotion activities. Research reviews provide practitioners with an alternative means of keeping up to date with research developments at a reduced individual cost. However, traditional methods of reviewing research have been criticized for their lack of scientific rigour (Mulrow, 1987).

In order to overcome the limitations of traditional reviews, a more systematic approach to conducting reviews has been proposed (Mulrow, 1994; Cook et al., 1995; Chalmers and Altman, 1995). Systematic reviews, such as those conducted by the Cochrane Collaboration (Chalmers and Altman, 1995), involve the use of explicit criteria for study inclusion, explicit criteria for assessment of study quality and rigorous methods of data analysis and synthesis. Systematic reviews can be extended to include a statistical summarizing of results (Peto, 1987; Cook et al., 1995). Such reviews, known as *meta-analyses,* provide statistical information on whether a health intervention investigated in a number of studies has produced a health benefit. Given the capacity of systematic reviews to synthesize the findings of multiple research studies, such reviews are considered to represent a higher quality of research evidence than single, well-designed, randomized controlled trials.

Practice guidelines

Practice guidelines are systematically prepared statements of recommended care that enable practitioners and clients to make more appropriate health care decisions and are therefore intended to lead to the achievement of better health outcomes (Institute of Medicine, 1990; Sox and Woolf, 1993). Research evidence evaluating the efficacy of practice guidelines suggests that such an objective can be achieved (Grimshaw and Russell, 1993).

Whereas the development of practice guidelines in the past has primarily been based on the collection of expert opinions, more recently developed guidelines have been based on a critical appraisal of research evidence. This recent development has occurred as expert opinion has been shown to not always reflect the current state of knowledge, resulting in delays in the introduction of effective interventions and the withdrawal of ineffective or harmful interventions (Antman *et al.*, 1992).

Two examples of guidelines that are of particular relevance to health promotion have been the Canadian Guide to Clinical Preventive Health Care (Canadian Taskforce on the Periodic Health Examination, 1994) and the Guide to Clinical Preventive Services (US Preventive Services Taskforce, 1996). For each preventive activity considered by these guidelines, a recommendation for use is made using a five-point scale. Those activities considered capable of providing a benefit are classified as either A or B. Those proven to be ineffective or harmful, D or E. Those interventions where there is insufficient evidence of either benefit or harm are classified as C. Recommendations of the Canadian Taskforce regarding tobacco-caused disease are shown in Table 8.2.

Although research evidence provides the basis for the development of practice guidelines, the potential health, social and economic consequence of each recommendation necessitates the consideration of additional information. Additional factors considered in the development of the Canadian and US guidelines included: the burden of suffering of a particular health issue; the availability of professional expertise and technology; intervention costs; the potential for intervention harm; medico-legal issues; intervention remuneration; and intervention compliance (Canadian Taskforce on the Periodic Health Examination, 1994; Sox and Woolf, 1993). Practice guidelines therefore provide an example of how research evidence can and

Table 8.2 Guidelines concerning prevention of tobacco-caused disease (Source: Canadian Taskforce, 1994)

Recommendation

There is good evidence to support counselling for smoking cessation for individuals who smoke (*A level recommendation*). Nicotine replacement therapy can be effective as an adjunct (*A level Recommendation*).

There is fair evidence to support referral to other programmes after offering smoking cessation advice (*B level recommendation*).

There is fair evidence to support counselling to prevent smoking initiation for adolescents (*B level recommendation*). Educational programmes have not been shown to significantly reduce tobacco initiation. Counselling by physicians to prevent smoking initiation has not been evaluated but given the burden of illness, the benefits of preventing addiction, the effectiveness of other smoking-related counselling, and the support of expert opinion, all children and adolescents should be counselled on avoiding tobacco use.

There is insufficient evidence to evaluate counselling to reduce environmental tobacco smoke exposure (*C level recommendation*), but it may be useful to combine such counselling with cessation advice, again based on the burden of suffering, the potential benefits of the intervention and the effectiveness of cessation advice.

Given the magnitude of the problem, educational programmes, counselling and healthy public policies are all vital.

---

needs to be integrated with additional information to inform health promotion policy and decision making.

The Canadian and US guidelines focus on the provision of preventive care interventions in primary health care settings. Currently no equivalent guidelines exist for the conduct of health promotion interventions in settings such as schools, work places and other community settings. The development of such guidelines is an important priority for health promotion if it is to improve its relevance as a means of enhancing the health of the community.

THE STAGED APPROACH TO HEALTH PROMOTION: A FRAMEWORK FOR SYSTEMATICALLY APPLYING RESEARCH EVIDENCE TO THE PRACTICE OF HEALTH PROMOTION

The Staged Approach to Health Promotion details a logical sequence of questions that guide health promotion practitioners when deciding which health promotion initiatives to undertake (Sanson-Fisher and Campbell, 1994). Reference to research evidence when answering each of these questions provides a structured mechanism whereby such evidence can be explicitly and systematically incorporated into the routine planning and conduct of health promotion initiatives.

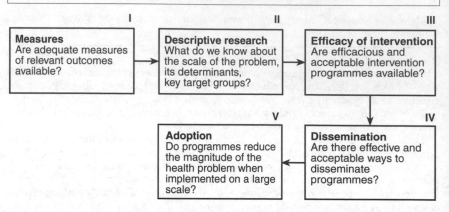

Figure 8.1 The Staged Approach to Health Promotion model (Sanson-Fisher and Campbell, 1994; reproduced by permission of the *Health Promotion Journal of Australia*).

When applying the model, the practitioner determines whether sufficient research evidence is available to answer the questions posed by each stage. Where sufficient evidence is available, the nature of the evidence guides the choice and design of the health promotion initiative to be undertaken. If insufficient evidence is available concerning a particular health issue, the practitioner may choose another issue as a focus for their activity. Alternatively, and where feasible in terms of access to skills and resources, the practitioner may elect to collect research data to redress the identified deficiency in evidence. The Staged Approach to Health Promotion consists of five sequential stages, described in Figure 8.1 and discussed in more detail in the following sections.

Stage 1: Adequacy of measures

The first stage of the model involves the health promotion practitioner asking whether accurate measurement techniques are available to assess the health status of a population and the outcomes of health promotion interventions. To answer these questions, the practitioner needs to critically appraise available research evidence to determine whether existing measures are:

- *reliable* (estimates the extent of the health issue consistently over time, place and between practitioners);
- *valid* (measures what it intends to measure);
- *acceptable* to consumers (cost, time, ease, sensitivity);
- *sensitive* to detect small differences in risk.

An individual's self-report is the most commonly used measure of smoking status, the reliability and validity of which have been assessed in numerous studies (Velicer *et al.*, 1992). The accuracy of self-reported smoking status varies considerably, with the greatest extent of inaccuracy occurring in those situations where there are high pressures to report not being a smoker (Velicer *et al.*, 1992). The value of all subsequent decisions and actions of the practitioner – such as the identification of the need for intervention (the number of smokers), identification of those with the most need for intervention (the group with the most smokers) and demonstration of an improvement in health status (intervention efficacy) – is dependent upon the selection of an adequate measure at this stage.

Stage 2: Descriptive research

In the second stage, the practitioner asks a series of questions directed at obtaining information that will aid in the targeting and design of intervention programmes. The particular questions concern:

- *the magnitude of the health issue (prevalence, incidence)*. Evidence concerning the relative burden of suffering imposed on the community by different health issues is required to ensure that practitioners focus their initiatives on those issues that have the capacity to provide the greatest health gain;
- *which population groups experience the greatest burden of illness*. Evidence identifying the population groups with the greatest burden of suffering is required so that initiatives can address those groups with the greatest need for intervention. Particular factors of interest include age, gender, ethnicity and socioeconomic status. Macfarlane and Jamrozik (1993) reported that differentials in smoking prevalence between males in blue and white-collar occupations increased between 1984 and 1991, an increase attributed to a more marked reduction in smoking among white-collar males than among those in blue-collar occupations. Without an understanding of such data, practitioners are less likely to address those groups with the greatest need for intervention and thus are more likely to exacerbate existing differentials in health status;
- *the perceived determinants of the health issue*. Quantitative and qualitative evidence is required to identify the individual, social and environmental factors associated with the development of health issues and the factors that act as barriers to the remediation of such issues. These factors include an individual's knowledge of health risks and their consequences, their attitudes and beliefs about health risks and behavioural skills in avoiding health risks. In addition, social and structural factors such as income, accessibility of health-damaging products and access to appropriate health care services also need to be considered. Research evidence has demonstrated that despite the existence of laws

prohibiting the sale of tobacco products to children, compliance with such laws is limited (Centers for Disease Control, 1990; Thomas and Toffler, 1990; Sanson-Fisher et al., 1992). An understanding of such a factor is required if health promotion practitioners are to focus their interventions on the most important determinants of, or barriers to changing a health issue;

● *the social and institutional settings through which population groups can be accessed.* Evidence is required to identify those locations where: those groups most in need of intervention can be most effectively reached; interventions have been demonstrated to be both appropriate and acceptable; and where interventions have been effective in producing a health benefit. Possible settings for accessing population subgroups include schools, work places, health care providers, recreational organizations and through the media. Without an understanding of where best to access a target population, health promotion practitioners may expend scarce health promotion resources on undertaking interventions in settings where the likelihood of achieving health benefits is limited.

Stage 3: Efficacy

This stage is concerned with the practitioner asking whether particular health promotion interventions can change the magnitude of a health issue under ideal circumstances (programme efficacy). In answering this question, practitioners should consider, together with the hierarchy of evidence discussed previously, whether a reported evaluation:

1. has a clearly defined and testable question;
2. includes a full description of the intervention;
3. details the validity and reliability of all the measures;
4. measures relevant outcome measures;
5. includes relevant process measures (utilization, acceptability, adherence);
6. includes an economic analysis.

Efficacy studies can vary in size and complexity. The majority of efficacy studies concerning smoking uptake or cessation involve the implementation of interventions conducted in single settings such as in general practice (Kottke et al., 1988; Glynn et al., 1990; Mattick and Baillie, 1992). Efficacy studies may also involve multifactorial intervention designs applied to large populations in a number of geographically defined areas (Green and Kreuter, 1991; CART Project Team, 1996a).

Difficulties in conducting rigorous large-scale community-based trials have been illustrated by a number of reviews (Donner et al., 1990; CART

Project Team, 1997). In one review, 13 studies were identified that had a focus on preventing either cardiovascular disease or cancer (CART Project Team, 1997). None of the 13 studies was assessed as meeting standard criteria defining a research design of adequate quality.

The COMMIT project, one of two studies judged to be most methodologically adequate (CART Project Team, 1997), evaluated the effect on smoking rates of interventions in 11 Canadian and United States communities (COMMIT Research Group, 1995a,b). No difference was observed between control and intervention communities in smoking cessation rates for heavy smokers, the focus of the intervention. However, a greater cessation rate among light to moderate smokers was observed in the intervention communities (COMMIT Research Group, 1995a,b). No difference in the decrease in community prevalence of smoking was evident between intervention and control communities. These modest findings, together with those from other community-based interventions, suggest that this intervention approach has yet to live up to its promise in providing health benefits to communities (Susser, 1995).

Without an understanding of the efficacy of health promotion interventions, particularly community-wide interventions, the health promotion practitioner is less likely to select and implement an intervention approach that has a capacity to achieve a health benefit and less likely to do so cost-effectively.

Stage 4: Dissemination trials

If research evidence has demonstrated the efficacy of an intervention approach, the next task of the health promotion practitioner is to determine whether such programmes have been demonstrated by research to be effective when implemented under real-world conditions (programme effectiveness). In order for interventions to be effective, they need to be effectively distributed, accepted and adopted by health promotion practitioners or agents and, as a result, contribute to improvements in health status. In determining the effectiveness of an intervention, the health promotion practitioner should consider the same study design and quality criteria as described previously for determining the efficacy of an intervention.

Although, health promotion research focusing on the dissemination of interventions has been limited (Orlandi et al., 1990; National Health Strategy, 1993; Oldenburg et al., 1996) the need for this form of research evidence is clear. Copeman et al. (1989) reported that 12 months after purchasing an efficacious smoking cessation programme, only 47% of general practitioners reported using it. Each practitioner recruited an average of 6.7 smokers to the programme, which represented 7% of the eligible smokers. Only 25–30% of patients who were told of the programme commenced it. Twenty-four percent of the participating patients reported that they had stopped smoking.

Without an understanding of how well an intervention is likely to be adopted by health promotion practitioners and agents in the community and how effective it is under these conditions, the health promotion practitioner is unlikely to select an intervention that has the potential to achieve desired health goals.

Stage 5: Adoption

The task for the health promotion practitioner in this final stage is to determine whether interventions demonstrated to be efficacious and effective have been adopted on a widespread basis by health agencies at the local, state and national level. Where such an adoption has occurred, the health promotion practitioner needs to establish whether the intervention has reduced the magnitude of the target health problem, risk or need.

Having adopted an efficacious and effective intervention for implementation, regular evaluation monitoring of health outcomes is required. Such evaluation should address some of the factors described in Stage 2 of the model to determine whether change in health status has occurred. If such evaluation indicates the absence of a sustained effect, the task of the health promotion practitioner is to develop modifications to the intervention or to identify new intervention approaches.

The application of the Staged Approach to Health Promotion emphasizes the importance of identifying appropriate evidence in each stage as a basis for moving to the next. Given the large costs associated with the widespread implementation of an intervention programme, the quality of the evidence and the proficiency of the critical appraisal and decision-making processes in the early stages of the model are central to whether health promotion activities selected in the later stages will contribute to improving the health of the community.

BARRIERS TO THE PRACTICE OF EVIDENCED-BASED HEALTH PROMOTION

There are a number of possible barriers to the practice of evidence-based health promotion. These include: a lack of quality research evidence; a lack of funding for health promotion research and evaluation; a lack of training and consequently of practitioner skills in data collection and critical appraisal; difficulties in conducting health promotion research in accordance with biomedical models of research; and a lack of acceptance of evidence-based practice as being relevant to health promotion.

Lack of quality research evidence

Relative to other areas of health-related research, there is a limited tradition and amount of quality research addressing best practice in health promotion (National Health Strategy, 1993). Equally, the practice of health promotion has not generally incorporated a focus on rigorously evaluating the efficacy and effectiveness of health promotion initiatives. In those instances where health promotion initiatives have been evaluated, the results of such evaluations are infrequently reported.

One consequence is that relatively limited research evidence is available upon which the health promotion practitioner can make an informed decision regarding the focus for their practice. Reviews of intervention efficacy and effectiveness in a number of health promotion areas also reveal that the quality of the available research evidence is frequently not of a sufficient standard upon which to make an informed decision (NHS Centre for Reviews and Dissemination, 1996; CART Project Team, 1997; Heaney and Goetzel, 1997).

Lack of funding

A further barrier to the practice of evidence-based health promotion concerns the system and level of health promotion research/evaluation funding. The allocation of funds to health promotion research in the past has been inadequate. A review of funding allocations by the National Health and Medical Research Council of Australia (Sanson-Fisher, 1985) indicated that 3.9% of research funds were allocated to health promotion research. Although this deficiency was recognized by the establishment of funding for public health research separate from that for biomedical research, support for public health research remains relatively limited, accounting for approximately 6.3% of the total research monies allocated (National Health and Medical Research Council, 1995).

Funding of health promotion research has traditionally been based on a *laissez-faire* approach where the interests of the researcher are the principal determinants of the focus and type of research that is undertaken (Doherty, 1982). Given that funding for health promotion research or practice is unlikely to increase significantly in the foreseeable future, one possible means of increasing the amount of quality research evidence is to adopt a targeted or mission-orientated approach to funding health promotion research (Fredrickson, 1981; Doherty, 1982).

In a targeted funding approach, a specific health promotion issue is selected by a government or agency, which then either seeks proposals for research initiatives addressing this issue or directs agency staff to focus their activities on it. In addition to specifying the focus of activity, the type of research (measures, descriptive, efficacy, dissemination) could also be specified. In this way, the amount and quality of evidence to be gained from existing funding could be maximized as a basis for determining future health promotion initiatives (National Health Strategy, 1993).

Lack of practitioner skill

If health promotion practitioners are unaware of or do not have the skills to practise evidence-based health promotion, it is extremely unlikely that such an approach to practice will flourish. The practice of evidence-based health promotion is founded in part upon a practitioner having the skills to collect data and critically appraise the research literature, which are in turn dependent upon knowledge and skill in both epidemiology and bio-statistics. For health promotion practitioners to acquire such knowledge and skills, they need to be essential components of all undergraduate and postgraduate health promotion training programmes. This is not currently the case.

Difficulties in conducting high-quality health promotion research

A further possible barrier to the conduct of evidence-based health promotion concerns the relative difficulty of conducting research that is of a sufficient quality and has the capacity to assess the objectives of health promotion. An inflexible application of the essentially biomedical hierarchy of research evidence will limit the practice of evidence-based health promotion as the stated criteria of evidence quality do not reflect the practical and design issues involved in undertaking population-based research (Koepsell et al., 1991).

The conduct of large-scale community-based trials, a necessary step in disseminating efficacious health promotion interventions, demonstrates the difficulties associated with the application of randomized controlled designs to population-based health promotion research (Farquar et al., 1985; Puska et al., 1985). Difficulties associated with such research include: the establishment of adequate and sufficient numbers of communities as controls in intervention research; determining an appropriate sample of individuals and communities allowing for clustered sample designs; and accounting for community sampling in analyses (Donner et al., 1990; CART Project Team, 1996a). In addition to such research design issues, particular difficulties in conducting scientifically rigorous community-based trials include the cost of implementation, feasibility issues and analytical limitations. Despite these difficulties, a capacity exists for the development of new and modified research solutions that enable the objectives of both health promotion and evidence-based practice to be met (Susser, 1995; CART Project Team, 1996a).

Lack of acceptance of the relevance of evidence-based practice to health promotion

Considerable resistance exists to the adoption of an evidence-based approach to professional practice (Grahame-Smith, 1995; Sackett *et al.*, 1996; Tutt, 1996; Anonymous, 1996). Much of this resistance appears to stem from the view that evidence-based practice is derived from the dominant biomedical paradigm of health care delivery, a paradigm that places an emphasis on physical intervention to remedy a manifest disease in individuals, rather than interventions that have a social, holistic and population focus on health. Such a paradigm is also perceived to be characterized by a concept of science that emphasizes empirical research methods, methods that do not always lend themselves to the analysis of the social determinants and dimensions of health (Anonymous, 1996). In this context, the adoption of evidence-based practice may be seen to reflect a further medicalization of health, whereby the values and methods of medical science are used to solve community and social health problems (Illich, 1975).

Evidence-based health promotion does not involve a dependence upon research evidence as a basis for decision making. In contrast, it requires that the biomedical values and methods inherent in its advocacy of research evidence are balanced by consideration of a variety of community, professional, political and economic issues. Similarly, evidence-based health promotion recognizes the reality of political or other circumstances precluding the application of an evidence-based approach in some instances. Finally, evidence-based health promotion practice does not preclude action if research evidence of the highest quality is not available.

Evidence-based health promotion therefore promotes a balanced approach to practice which emphasizes and extends the responsibility of the health promotion practitioner in deciding the focus and form of health promotion activity. In proposing that health promotion practitioners systematically consider research evidence in decision-making, the challenge for the practitioner is not so much the adoption of a contrasting paradigm of action but of a balanced consideration of evidence from a number of sources. Evidence-based health promotion therefore requires that the value of both research evidence and evidence derived from other sources be subject to critical appraisal.

CONCLUSION

Evidence-based health promotion involves the systematic integration of research evidence into the planning and implementation of health promotion activities. It has been argued that the incorporation of such an approach could result in greater health gains for the community. For health promotion to meet the challenge of providing an enhanced role for research evidence in its decision making, significant improvements in health promotion research and training are required. In addition, if health promotion is to further develop its role as a vehicle for improving the health of the community, a need exists for practitioners to adopt a balanced and critical approach to their decision-making. The Staged Approach to Health promotion represents one model that can be applied by health promotion practitioners to aid such a critical approach to their practice.

REFERENCES

Anonymous. (1996) How effective are effectiveness reviews? *Health Education Journal*, **55**, 359–362.

Antman, E., Lau, I., Kupelnick, B., Masteller, F. and Chalmers, T. (1992) A comparison of results of meta-analyses of randomised control trials and recommendations of clinical experts. *Journal of the American Medical Association*, **268**, 240–248.

Canadian Taskforce on the Periodic Health Examination. (1994) *The Canadian Guide to Clinical Preventive Health Care*. Canada Communication Group.

CART Project Team. (1996a) Developing methodologies for evaluating community-wide health promotion. *Health Promotion International*, **11**(3), 227–235.

CART Project Team. (1997) Community action for health promotion: A review of methods and outcomes 1990–1995. *American Journal of Preventive Medicine*. (in press).

Centers for Disease Control. (1990) Cigarette sales to minors – Colorado, 1989. *Journal of the American Medical Association*. **264**, 2734.

Chalmers, I. and Altman, D. (1995) *Systematic Reviews*, London: BMJ Publishing.

COMMIT Research Group. (1995a) Community Intervention Trial for Smoking Cessation (COMMIT). I. Cohort results from a four-year community intervention. *American Journal of Public Health*, **85**(2), 183–192.

COMMIT Research Group. (1995b) Community Intervention Trial for Smoking Cessation (COMMIT). II. Changes in adult cigarette smoking prevalence. *American Journal of Public Health*, **85**(2), 193–200.

Cook, D. Sackett, O. and Spitzer, W. (1995) Methodological guidelines for systematic reviews of randomised control trials in health care from the Potsdam Consultation on Meta-Analysis. *Journal of Clinical Epidemiology*, **48**, 167–171.

Copeman, R., Swannell, R., Pincus, D. and Woodhead, K. (1989) Utilisation of the smokescreen smoking cessation programme by general practitioners and their patients. *Medical Journal of Australia*, **151**, 83–87.

Covell, D., Uman, G. and Manning, P. (1985) Information needs in office practice: are they being met? *Annals of Internal Medicine*, **103**, 596–599.

Davis, D., Thomson, M., Oxman, A. and Haynes, R. (1995) Changing physician performance. A systematic review of the effect of continuing medical education strategies. *Journal of the American Medical Association*, **274**, 700–705.

Doherty, R. (1982) Follow the yellow brick road: medical research policy in the land of Oz. *Medical Journal of Australia*, **1**, 199–203.

Donner. A., Brown, K. and Brasher, P. (1990) A methodological review of non-therapeutic intervention trials employing cluster randomization, 1979–1989. *International Journal of Epidemiology*, **19**, 795–800.

Downie, R., Tannahill, C. and Tannahill, A. (1996) *Health Promotion: Models and Value*, Oxford: Oxford University Press.

Evans, C., Haynes, R., Birkett, N. *et al.* (1996) Does a mailed continuing education program improve clinician performance? Results of a randomised trial in antihypertensive care. *Journal of the American Medical Association*, **255**, 501–504.

Farquar, J., Fortmann, S., Maccoby, N. *et al.* (1985) The Stanford Five-City Project: design and methods. *American Journal of Epidemiology*, **122**, 323–334.

Flay, B. (1986) Efficacy and effectiveness trials (and other phases of research) in the development of health promotion programs. *Preventive Medicine*, **15**, 451–474.

Fleming, M., Barry, K.L., Manwell, L., Johnson, K. and London, R. (1997) Brief physician advice for problem alcohol drinker. *Journal of the American Medical Association*, **277**, 1039–1045.

Fredrickson, D. (1981) Biomedical research in the 1980s. *New England Journal of Medicine* **304**, 509–517.

Glanz, K., Lewis, F. and Rimer, B. (1996) *Health Behavior and Health Education: Theory, Research, and Practice*, 2nd edn, San Francisco, CA: Jossey-Bass.

Glynn, T., Boyd, G. and Gruman, J. (1990) Essential elements of self-help/minimal intervention strategies for smoking cessation. *Health Education Quarterly*, **17**, 329–345.

Grahame-Smith, D. (1995) Evidence based medicine: Socratic dissent. *British Medical Journal*, **310**, 1126–1127.

Green, L. and Kreuter, M. (1991) *Health Promotion Planning: An Educational and Environmental Approach*, Mountain View, CA: Mayfield.

Grimshaw, J. and Russell, I. (1993) Effect of clinical guidelines on medical practice: a systematic review of rigorous evaluations. *Lancet*, **342**, 1317–1322.

Haynes. R., Davis, D., McKibbon, A. and Tugwell, P. (1984) A critical appraisal of the efficacy of continuing medical education. *Journal of the American Medical Association*, **251**, 61–64.

Heaney, C. and Goetzel, R. (1997) A review of health-related outcomes of multi-component worksite health promotion programs. *American Journal of Health Promotion*, **11**(4). 290–308.

Illich, I. (1975) *Medical Nemesis. The Exploration of Health*, London: Calder and Boyars Ltd.

Institute of Medicine. (1990) *Clinical Practice Guidelines: Directions for a New Program*, (eds M. Field and K. Lohr), Washington DC: Institute of Medicine, National Academy Press.

Koepsell, T., Martin, D., Diehr, P. *et al.* (1991) Data analysis and sample size issues in evaluation of community based health promotion and disease prevention programs: a mixed model analysis of variance approach. *Journal of Clinical Epidemiology*, **44**, 701–713.

Kottke, T., Battista, R., DeFriese, G. and Brekke, M. (1988) Attributes of successful smoking cessation interventions in medical practice: a meta-analysis of 39 controlled trials. *Journal of the American Medical Association*, **259**, 2882–2889.

Last, M. (1995) *A Dictionary of Epidemiology*. Oxford: Oxford University Press.

Macfarlane, J. and Jamrozik, K. (1993) Tobacco in Western Australia: patterns of smoking among adults from 1974 to 1991. *Australian Journal of Public Health* **17**, 350–358.

Maclean, H. and Eakin, J. (1992) Health promotion research methods: expanding the repertoire. *Canadian Journal of Public Health*, **83** (supp) 1.

Mattick, R. and Baillie, A. (1992) *An Outline of Approaches to Smoking Cessation*. Canberra: Australian Government Publishing Service.

Mulrow, C. (1987) The medical review article: state of science. *Annals of Internal Medicine*, **106**(3), 458–488.

Mulrow, C. (1994) Rationale for systematic reviews. *British Medical Journal*, **309**, 597–599.

National Health and Medical Research Council. (1995) *Clinical Practice Guidelines – The Management of Early Breast Cancer*. Canberra: Australian Government Publishing Service.

National Health Strategy. (1993) *Pathways to Better Health*, Canberra: Australian Government Publishing Service.

NHS Centre for Reviews and Dissemination. (1996) *Review of the Research on the Effectiveness of Health Service Interventions to Reduce Variations in Health: Part I.* York: NHS Centre for Reviews and Dissemination.

Nutbeam, D., Smith, C. and Catford, J. (1990) Evaluation in health education: a review of progress, possibilities and problems. *Journal of Epidemiology and Community Health* **4**, 83–89.

Nutbeam, D., Wise, M., Bauman, A., Harris, E. and Leeder, S. (1993) *Goals and Targets for Australia's Health in the Year 2000 and Beyond*, Sydney: Department of Public Health, University of Sydney.

Oldenburg, B., Hardcastle, D. and French, M. (1996) How does research contribute to evidence-based practice in health promotion? *Health Promotion Journal of Australia*, **6**(2), 15–20.

Orlandi, M., Landers, C., Weston, R. and Haley, N. (1990) Diffusion of health promotion innovations. In K. Glanz, F. Lewis and B. Rimer (eds) *Health Behaviors and Health Education: Theory, Research and Practice*, San Francisco, CA: Jossey-Bass.

Peto, R. (1987) Why do we need systematic overviews of randomised trials? *Statistics in Medicine*, **6**, 233–241.

Puska, P., Missinen, A., Tuomilehto, J. *et al.* (1985) The community-based strategy to prevent coronary heart disease: conclusions from the ten years of the North Karelia Project. *Annual Review of Public Health*, **6**, 147–193.

Ramsey, P., Carline, J., Inui, T. *et al.* (1991) Changes over time in the knowledge base of practicing internists. *Journal of the American Medical Association* **266**, 1103–1107.

Redman, S. (1996) Towards a research strategy to support public health programs for behaviour change. *Australian and New Zealand Journal of Public Health*, **20**(4), 352–358.

Rosenberg, W. and Donald, A. (1995) Evidence based medicine: an approach to clinical problem-solving. *British Medical Journal*, **310**, 1122–1126.

Russell, M., Wilson, C., Taylor, C. and Baker, C. (1979) Effect of general practitioners' advice against smoking. *British Medical Journal*, **283**, 231–235.

Sackett, D., Rosenberg, W., Gray, J., Haynes, R. and Richardson, W. (1996) Evidence-based medicine: what it is and what it isn't. *British Medical Journal* **312**, 71–72.

Sackett, D., Richardson, W., Rosenberg, W. and Haynes, R. (1997) *Evidence-Based Medicine: How to Practise and Teach EBM*, Edinburgh: Churchill Livingstone.

Sanson-Fisher, R. (1985) Commentary: behavioural science and its relation to medicine – a need for positive action. *Community Health Studies* **9**(3), 275–283.

Sanson-Fisher, R. and Campbell, E. (1994) Health research in Australia – its role in achieving the goals and targets. *Health Promotion Journal of Australia*, **4**(3), 28–33.

Sanson-Fisher, R., Schofield, M. and See, M. (1992) Availability of cigarettes to minors. *Australian Journal of Public Health* **16**(4), 354–359.

Sibley, J., Sackett, D., Newfeld, V. *et al.* (1982) A randomised trial of continuing medical education. *New England Journal of Medicine* **306**, 511–515.

Sox, H. and Woolf, S. (1993) Evidence-based practice guidelines from the US Preventive Services Task Force. *Journal of the American Medical Association*, **269**(20), 2678.

Susser, M. (1995) Editorial: the tribulations of trials intervention in communities. *American Journal of Public Health*, **85**(2), 156–164.

Thomas, B. and Toffler, W. (1990) The illegal sale of cigarettes to minors in Oregon. *Journal of Family Practice* **31**, 206–208.

Tutt, D. (1996) How useful is research evidence to practitioners? *Health Promotion Journal of Australia* **6**(2), 32–36.

US Preventive Services Taskforce. (1996) *Guide to Clinical Preventive Services*, Baltimore: Williams and Wilkins.

Velicer, W., Prochaska, J. Rossi, J. and Snow, M. (1992) Assessing outcome in smoking cessation studies. *Psychological Bulletin*, **111**, 23–41.

Winett, R. (1995) A framework for health promotion and disease prevention programs. *American Psychologist*, **50**(5), 341–350.

Woolf, S., Battista. R., Anderson, G., Logan, A., Wang, E. and the Canadian Taskforce on the Periodic Health Examination. (1990) Assessing the clinical effectiveness of preventive manoeuvres: analytic principles and systematic methods in reviewing evidence and developing clinical practice recommendations. *Journal of Clinical Epidemiology*, **43**, 891–905.

| 9 | **Ethics and evaluating health promotion** |

David Scott

Much has been written about the ethics of health promotion (cf. Seed-house, 1986, 1988), but as yet very little about the ethics of evaluation. One of the reasons for this is that evaluation is considered to be about the dispassionate collection of data and that its justification is therefore epistemological rather than ethical. That is, it is concerned with giving accounts of health promotion projects which enable evaluators to come to certain definite conclusions about how best to go about improving health in the community. This view has been challenged recently by the advocacy of evaluation paradigms which stress the need for formative as opposed to summative judgements, which argue that nomothetic conceptions of research/evaluation[1] fail to account for the complexity of human affairs they seek to describe, and which understand knowledge as tentative, speculative and contextualized (cf. Simons, 1984, 1987; Norris, 1990).

EXPERIMENTAL PROCEDURES

Two opposing paradigms will be explored in this chapter. The traditional view emphasizes the collection of facts about health promotion activities, stresses the capacity of evaluators to produce knowledge which can be generalized to other settings, both in place and time, and is judged by public and verifiable criteria. This is a monolinear view of knowledge and is empiricist[2] in orientation.The methodology adopted is invariably experimental and where, for practical reasons, experimental conditions cannot be created, quasi-experimental methods are used. With the latter, evaluators can be less sure of the validity and reliability of their conclusions.

There are some important consequences of this approach. The first is that it assumes a particular view of the theory–practice relationship. This has been called the technical-rationality model.[3] If theoretical statements about health promotion activities can be made and these statements prescribe appropriate actions for practitioners (those actions having been legitimized by the collection of data using experimental and quasi-experimental designs), it would seem irrational for them not to follow those precepts. The practitioner is here understood as a technician in thrall to the research community. Their job is faithfully to apply the principles and understanding developed by others. This represents a particular view of the relationship between theory and practice and implies a separation between them (see Carr and Kemmis, 1986; Carr, 1995, for the arguments against).

Secondly, it implies a particular view of ethical behaviour. Since the emphasis is placed on the adequacy of the description made and this encompasses other settings in time and place, to ignore such prescriptions would be unethical. This is regardless of the means used to come to such conclusions. We are thus confronted by the familiar dilemma of ends and means. If there are certain good ends, then the designation of means is purely a technical matter. The parameters of the debate are constructed by two ends of a spectrum; at one extreme there are a number of deontological theories (cf. Kant, 1974–1977) which centre on notions of duty, absolutism and the ascription of moral principles. Ends, however ethically justified, can never be the justification for means. Means have to be judged as ethically sound in their own right. At the other extreme, there are various forms of utilitarianism (cf. Mill, 1910), in which means are judged in terms of whether they lead to good ends. Utilitarians have difficulties in defining the greater good – whether this is understood as forms of pleasure or as some other designated benefit – but this view sanctions particular human suffering if it can be shown that, or predicted that, it will lead to the greater good of the community. The collection of authoritative knowledge about health education processes may be considered to be of this kind, in that ethical safeguards to govern the collection of data need not apply because research/evaluation will ultimately contribute to a better society.

INTERPRETIVE APPROACHES

The second evaluation paradigm understands the empirical process in a different way. Here the evaluator/researcher is considered to be an essential part of the collection of data. Their views and beliefs cannot be separated from the way they go about collecting data and thus from the analysis and synthesis of those data. Observations are understood as proceeding from particular theories about human behaviour and about how as human beings we can know reality. Human beings are understood as meaning-makers who are involved in interpretive activity during their lives. Social life therefore has to be understood in terms of the double hermeneutic (Giddens, 1984). There are two versions of this. In the first, human beings are conceptualized as interpretive actors who proceed on the basis of how they reconstruct their own and other people's actions. However, the data collector is in the same position, that is, they are also engaged in interpretive activity. Evaluators are therefore involved in making interpretations of the actions and beliefs of social actors who themselves are engaged in interpretive activity. The double hermeneutic here renders their accounts problematic.

However, there is a further version of the double hermeneutic which is significant for the way social life can be understood. Unlike in the natural sciences, researchers/evaluators' perceptions of human activity are, through various means, fed back to those social actors which has an effect on the interpretations they subsequently make. This renders the production of law-like and predictable accounts of human nature problematic. In short, this interpretive perspective may be distinguished from the positivist perspective of experimental and quasi-experimental researchers in the following ways: positivists argue that objective reality can be grasped; researchers can remain neutral with their values separate from the descriptions of reality they provide; observations and generalizations are asituational and atemporal; causality is linear; and enquiry is an objective activity (cf. Denzin, 1989). Interpretive evaluators understand the research process in a different way: ontology has to be understood as separate from epistemology or at least that which we can observe never unproblematically relates to those mechanisms, causal or otherwise, which ontologically underpin society (Bhaskar, 1979); researchers are an essential part of the research process with their values and preconceptions underpinning the data that they can collect; observations and generalizations are context specific; reasons as they are expressed by social actors can also function as causes; objectivity is a constructed notion (cf. Scott, 1996a). The effect of this is to designate knowledge in a different way from positivists. Knowledge is not understood as nomothetic but as speculative, informing, rich in depth and contextualized.

COVERT ETHICAL STANCES

The implications of this paradigm are profound in relation to ethics. Since the data gatherer is an essential part of the research process, how they behave – the ethical decisions they make – determines the type of data they collect. Here the epistemological and ethical aspects of the research process are closely tied together. Three models have been suggested. The first is covert evaluation. The evaluator does not inform participants in the evaluation that they are being evaluated because they wish to avoid reactivity. If participants in the evaluation know that they are taking part, then they are less likely to behave naturally. This way of acting applies to evaluation whether it is positioned within experimental, correlational or qualitative paradigms. Experimental researchers, for example, rarely inform members of control and experimental groups that they are taking part in an experiment and certainly do not make the distinction clear to participants. Much experimental work cannot avoid reactivity since its rationale is to control those important variables which in real life complicate the issue. It is therefore a deliberate artefact and, though this has implications for its ecological validity or ability to generalize to other settings which have not been constructed in the same way, proponents of experimental methods argue that this is the only way of actually testing propositions. This artificiality can be seen most clearly in the time frame it adopts. It is assumed that the effects of interventions will show up or not show up at the point of testing, whether this is immediate or later, and, further, that the full or completed effects of that intervention will manifest themselves at these points in time. In much experimental work, hypotheses are confirmed or disconfirmed on this basis and yet health promotion messages are frequently complex in their effects and in how they influence behaviour (cf. Tones et al., 1994). Thus, experimentalists sacrifice some forms of ecological validity by the construction of artificial conditions, while at the same time (by using covert methods) they seek to enhance others.

If, on the other hand, it is conceded that participants in the evaluation construct the setting by their very presence (that, in other words, reactivity is an essential part of the process), then a different set of ethical parameters structure it. This refers to the fusion of horizons, a notion developed by Gadamer (1975) who argued that researchers inevitably approach research settings with a set of epistemological and ethical precepts by which they understand the world. Their approach is therefore always from within a tradition of understanding. These preunderstandings or prejudices fuse with the setting which they are interested in and this leads to the creation of new knowledge.

How does this interpretive view impact on ethical behaviour? One version accepts that evaluators bring to the evaluation setting a variety of prior ideas about the world, but assumes that they can bracket out this knowledge and thus construct reality without reference to their own beliefs and prejudgements. They are thus committed to present as full a picture of what is going on by referencing social actors' perceptions of reality. This is in essence the phenomenological approach.[4] Evaluators deliberately write themselves out of the picture and, more importantly they do everything in their power to present a full account, through participants' words, of that reality. In effect they deliberately diminish or conceal the reflexive element implicit in the evaluation process. This has implications for the power relationship between evaluator and evaluatee. Evaluators are denying (though this is of course theoretical and not real) their right to interpret the data they receive. They are therefore to some extent handing control of those data to participants in their evaluation. They are allowing those participants a veto over how their lives and activities are described in the evaluation report.

On the surface, this seems relatively straightforward. However, there are two major problems. First, each participant constructs their own account in terms of their knowledge of the circumstances in which that account is produced. Those circumstances might include how the participants understand what is expected of them and how that account will be received when it is inscribed in the text. It might be a deliberate response to the persona of the evaluator – much feminist research works on the assumption that only a woman, with her inbuilt sympathy can gather authentic data about other women (cf. Reinharz, 1992). Accounts, therefore, are always in effect presentations. Second, this phenomenological perspective assumes unjustifiably that participants have full knowledge of the perspectives that underpin their everyday actions. If we accept this argument, then we also have to accept that social actors are not able to transcend the limitations of consciousness. This can be expressed in four ways: human beings do not have full knowledge of the settings which structure their activities; human beings cannot have knowledge of the unintended consequences of their actions because the translation of intention to fulfilment of project is never unproblematic, and furthermore, what actually happens is the consequence of the sum of a multitude of human projects which have unforeseen consequences; third, social actors may not be aware of unconscious forces which drive them towards projects which consciously they do not wish to complete; fourth, social actors operate with tacit knowledge which they are either unable to articulate or are unaware of as they go about their lives (cf. Bhaskar, 1989). I will return to the problems of the limitations of consciousness later, as this has direct implications for the act of doing evaluation and the ethical frameworks that are adopted.

DEMOCRATIC EVALUATION

The second model is democratic evaluation. Simons (1984) suggests that evaluation should be underpinned by five principles. First, it is incumbent on the researcher/evaluator to act impartially, that is, 'withhold their judgements' or suspend their own value positions in deciding on important matters concerning the design of the evaluation and use of data. They should thus represent a range of views. Second, participants should have control over the release of data at every stage of the proceedings: after each data collection session (the right to read and amend interview transcripts); after each report writing session (the right to change, either by including or excluding, information in the report); and at the dissemination stage (the right to control the release of the data in either its raw or organized form). Thus, the control mechanism should be a series of negotiations between the researcher/evaluator and participants in the project. The implicit assumption here is that negotiations can take place on an equal basis and would thus be concerned with the fairness, accuracy and relevancy of what is going to be reported; both evaluator and evaluatee have sufficient understanding of the dissemination process to act from an equal base and together to decide on what should be included in the report when it is placed in the public domain. Fourth, research and evaluation are not activities which should compel participation. Fifth, the researcher/evaluator is accountable not just to participants in the project, but also to other bodies with an interest in the information that has been collected. In short, five principles should be applied: phenomenological bracketing; equality of control of data; negotiated control mechanisms; consent; and accountability.

I have already suggested two reasons why this approach is flawed: respondents construct accounts in terms of their understanding of the context in which the evaluation is taking place and purely phenomenological perspectives ignore the limitations of consciousness. However, the principal flaw is that, to borrow Habermas' (1978) concept of the 'ideal speech situation' which is essentially a fictive notion, data for an evaluation cannot be collected in ideal circumstances. This is not to deny the potential rationality inherent in good evaluation, but to suggest that in real life only a limited form of rationality can exist. This is because those factors which militate against the ideal of a free, open and uncoerced exchange of views are ever present in evaluation settings, constructed as they are in terms of vested interests, inadequate exchanges of information and differential amounts of power between participants, be they sponsors, managers, participants or other stakeholders. As Norris (1990: 134) suggests, the ideal speech situation is:

  a regulative idea (in the Kantian sense) which manifestly cannot be realized under present conditions, but which holds out the prospect of a genuine dialogue – an uncoerced exchange of differing arguments and viewpoints – from which truth might yet emerge at the end of the enquiry.

In addition, the deliberate bracketing out of the values of the evaluator so that they operate from a set of values which is universal in orientation (no evaluator can of course operate in an ethical vacuum) and which represents something which transcends the limited and everyday perspective of the evaluator (in effect, a god's eye view of reality) is not a practical possibility. This position, of course, does not rule out the possibility of adopting a reflexive posture in which those relevant values which drive the research at every moment and at every stage are identified and inscribed in some form or another in the report. Likewise, as I have suggested, negotiated control mechanisms and indeed negotiated processes of deciding which data are to be collected, how they are to be collected and inscribed cannot be achieved, but serve, in Norris' words, as 'a regulative ideal'. The evaluator, in short, always understands the consequences of the release of data into the public domain better than participants in the evaluation, though of course their understanding may be incomplete.

However, if evaluation is to be understood as democratic and contextualized, as focused on the particular health promotion intervention and as a means of correction to the ongoing programme, then a different rationale for evaluation and a different set of ethical and epistemological precepts apply. The evaluation is now considered to be formative and directed towards good practice in the particular circumstances of the evaluation. Though accounts of processes are provided, these cannot be generalized unproblematically from the case being evaluated to other cases, whether they are located in the present or are yet to be constructed by health promoters. Knowledge of health promotion activities is thus construed in a different way. The traditional approach (cf. Campbell and Stanley, 1963; Bracht and Glass, 1968) uses four criteria by which researchers can judge whether generalizability can be achieved or, in other words, whether the experimental findings apply to larger populations or other settings. These are: sound internal validity, credible external validity, reliability and objectivity. Educational evaluators have sought to distance themselves from this style of evaluation and substitute four different notions: credibility, transferability, dependability and confirmability. These have the effect of diluting the principle of generalized and absolutely verifiable knowledge, but their proponents argue that their descriptions of reality are now firmly rooted in the actual processes by which health promoters go about their business.

These four notions, developed by Guba and Lincoln (1985), have been criticized on two grounds. First, they are still located within a positivist framework. In effect, they make a number of assumptions about how the world can be known and what it is that is shared by positivists. For example, descriptions of health promotion activities and the theories subsequently developed from them represent in an unproblematic way what is and has actually happened. This approach has been called naive realism[5] and ignores textual and reflexive elements central to the research process as it is understood by interpretive researchers. Second, Hammersley (1992) has criticized the distinction between internal validity – those criteria internal to the experimental design which determine whether the observations made reflect the impact of the intervention or have been caused by other factors – and external validity – those criteria external to the experiment which allow judgements to be made about the generaliz- ability of the findings from the experimental sample to the larger popula- tion it represents – as incoherent because the one implies the other. If, therefore, the new model is based on the old which, it is suggested, is flawed, this simply compounds the original difficulty.

However, these four notions – credibility, transferability, dependability and confirmability – are qualitatively different because they acknowledge: a different relationship between the knower (or evaluator) and what they are seeking to describe; and the proper ascription of the relationship between the experimental case and the larger population – which is that it is tentative and speculative rather than certain. (This is because even if it is possible to operationalize variables, that operationalizing always involves a squeezing of reality to accommodate the demands of the mathe- matical model being constructed and that what is an appropriate set of variables depends on the making of certain assumptions before fieldwork takes place.)

Guba and Lincoln (1985) therefore want to replace the idea of internal validity – and its implicit assumption of representational realism – with one that takes account of multiple realities. That is, when they are evaluat- ing health promotion projects, practitioners may adopt different and conflicting perspectives which are equally valid. Evaluation needs to take account of this:

> The naturalist must show that he or she has represented those multi- ple constructions adequately, ... that the reconstructions ... that have been arrived at via the enquiry are credible to the constructors of the original multiple realities (Guba and Lincoln, 1985: 296).

Again, with respect to the second criterion used by experimental research- ers (external validity) they argue that:

> The naturalist cannot specify the external validity of an enquiry; he or she can provide only the thick description necessary to enable someone interested in making a transfer to reach a conclusion about whether the transfer can be contemplated as a possibility (Guba and Lincoln, 1985: 316).

Thus the burden of proof is placed firmly on the reader or user and this avoids the problem of treating the practitioner who uses the research evidence in order to design their own health promotion programmes as merely a technician in thrall to the research community (see above).

The third element in experimental research is that of reliability. Guba and Lincoln (1985) want to replace this by a notion of dependability. Since implicit in the interpretative research paradigm is the emergent notion of design, evaluation teams which wish to conduct enquiries about health promotion settings independently are unlikely to come to the same conclusions. It is not that they are likely to come to conflicting conclusions, though this is possible, but that they will represent the setting in different ways. However, Guba and Lincoln (1985: 318) do not want to abandon altogether the possibility of independently checking the validity of the data collected and of the conclusions drawn from that data set. They therefore developed the notion of an auditor to determine both the evaluation's dependability and their fourth criterion, confirmability (this is intended to replace the notion of objectivity). The auditor would have a number of tasks, chief of which would be to:

> ascertain whether the findings are grounded in the data ... whether inferences based on the data are logical, whether the utility of the category system: its clarity, explanatory power and fit to the data are realistic, and finally the degree and incidence of inquirer bias (Guba and Lincoln, 1985: 318).

In response to criticisms made about their four criteria, Guba and Lincoln (1989) developed a further set of criteria, which do not have their origins in a positivist perspective. They describe these as authenticity criteria. The first is fairness, which they argue is central to all types of evaluation: equal consideration should be given to all the various perspectives of participants in the evaluation, despite their unequal positioning in the hierarchical structure of the setting being evaluated. The second is educative authenticity. Implicit in this notion is the idea that evaluation does not just involve the neutral collection of evidence about health promotion activities but that the act of evaluation, by virtue of what it is, changes, and is intended to change, both the health promotion initiative and participants' knowledge about it. An evaluation is valid, for example, when individual participants' understanding of other viewpoints is enhanced. There is thus a necessary formative element in any evaluation. Their third criterion is catalytic authenticity. Here, the evaluation is judged to have succeeded or not based on whether it has contributed to better decision making within the organization or project being evaluated. They are thus committed to an explicit action-orientated perspective. Their fourth criterion reinforces this notion by stressing the need for evaluators always to aim, as a result of their activities, at empowering participants to act in better ways. Earlier I referred to the implicit assumption made by evaluators working within traditional perspectives, which is that participants are treated as technicians in thrall to the research/evaluation community. Guba and Lincoln's four criteria are designed to redress the balance by focusing on action and the enablement of wise decision making in health promotion settings.

Democratic evaluators propose a highly idealized form of evaluation, in which two main purposes sit uneasily alongside each other. In the first place, they stress forms of external accountability which include the right to know by various public bodies and in the second place, they acknowledge that health education settings (these are understood in their widest sense and incorporate a variety of stakeholders) are hierarchically arranged and thus the publication of members' accounts is potentially dangerous. The implication of this is that the evaluator may have to filter out knowledge which could potentially harm participants, even if those dangers are not apparent to the participants themselves. Regardless of the forms of negotiation undertaken by the researcher and those being researched, an ideal speech situation cannot exist and thus ultimate responsibility for the release of information must stay firmly with the researcher/evaluator. This is so because social actors in time and space have different and conflicting levels of knowledge about the evaluation setting. In short, in order for evaluators to proceed, they have to take account of the power structures in which they are working and this involves the adoption of a critical action approach.

CRITICAL ACTION APPROACHES

This means both that knowledge of health education settings and promotions involves the making of judgements and that the ethical dimensions of the cases being investigated have to be carefully thought through. This chapter is concerned fundamentally with the latter (see Chapter 3 for a discussion of the former). However, the ethical precepts which are relevant to health work mirror the ethical dimensions of evaluating it. This is, of course, only if evaluation is located within an interpretive paradigm and understood as contextualized, interactive and formative. Seedhouse (1988) has developed a grid which is an attempt to balance the conflicting impulses occasioned by health work. He argues that the fundamental principle of using such a grid is that workers must:

> ...honestly seek to enable the enhancing potentials of people ... In other words, the grid can be used legitimately only by those who are consistently opposed to *dwarfing*, and devoted to the fight against it (*dwarfing* can mean either the deliberate attempt to diminish people or any diminishing which is unavoidable)' (Seedhouse, 1988: 140).

The grid itself has four layers. In the first are the 'central conditions' necessary for health promotion: respect persons equally, create autonomy, respect autonomy and serve needs before wants. In the second are those ethical precepts which originate in deontological theories which act to guide behaviour: promise keeping, beneficence, truth telling and minimizing harm. At the third level, reference is made to consequentialist theories of ethics (for example, rule-following utilitarianism) and they therefore relate to the effects of actions on other people living in the community. They are: the increase of individual good; the increase of self-good; the increase of the good of a particular group; and the increase of the social good. The final layer includes those ethical precepts which relate to external considerations. These imply a level of calculation by the moral agent acting as a health educator and they remind us that ethical decision making, whether in health promotion or its evaluation, involves speculative activity. These precepts are as follows: evaluating the effectiveness and efficiency of action; justifying actions in terms of external evidence; respecting the wishes and legal rights of others; accepting the idea that facts may be disputed; assessing the degree of certainty of the evidence on which action is taken; and taking into consideration existing codes of practice and risk factors involved.

It is important to understand that each layer of the grid is not independent but inter-related. In other words, it would be considered unwise to make decisions about health work without referring to all the layers of the grid. The second point is that such a framework avoids reference to lists of prescribed behaviours, because ethical precepts are complicated, cannot be reduced to a list of moral absolutes and fundamentally have to make reference to the context in which they are being applied.

Evaluation as it has been reconceptualized in this chapter brings it much closer to the activity of health promotion itself; that is, since evaluation has a necessary formative element and is not understood as producing prescriptive knowledge for health promoters, it necessarily becomes a part of the health promotion initiative, whether conducted by the health promoter or some external agency. The implication of this is that the ethical framework suggested by Seedhouse requires little modification if it is to be used by evaluators, because it is constructed with the same types of ethical dilemmas in mind. Knowledge of health promotion activities is not understood as separate from the creation of better health in communities and for individual social actors. Furthermore, judgements which are specifically ethical in orientation also have relevance to judgements which are specifically epistemological in orientation. The two are closely related.

ETHICAL DILEMMAS IN EVALUATING HEALTH PROMOTION ACTIVITIES

In constructing an ethical framework for evaluators, three factors need to be taken into consideration. The first is that it is impossible to construct a list of ethical absolutes because some of the subsequent obligations they impose on evaluators may conflict. Telling lies may be necessary to maintain confidentiality. Or, to take another example, the evaluator may feel that it is important to protect the interests of a participant in the project, even if that participant does not fully understand the necessity of doing so. Burgess (1984:197) writes that:

In these terms, fieldworkers are constantly engaged in taking decisions about ethical issues in both 'open' and 'closed' research; they are involved in arriving at some form of compromise, whereby the impossibility of seeking informed consent from everyone, of telling the truth all the time and of protecting everyone's interests is acknowledged.

The second factor has already been referred to and this is that health promotion settings are hierarchically arranged, which means that knowledge of health promotion activities, processes and effects is always subject to the different interests of different people in the organization. This means that the data collected are always presentations, which makes it difficult to assess the authenticity of those data. It is therefore important to understand data collection not as a neutral activity but as subject to the effects of different agendas operating within the hierarchical setting of the evaluation. These power plays apply equally to the relationship between the evaluator and participants in their evaluation.

The third element to be taken into account is that evaluation is inevitably of a moving process. Evaluators are engaged both in feedback to the project, which changes what it is they are examining, and the promotion of a particular set of ideas about health. They cannot avoid responsibility for the fact that their evaluation is driven by a particular view of health and that their agenda is normative; action that results from their efforts is always part of their brief.

Bearing in mind these three points, it is now possible to construct an ethical framework for evaluation which, let me repeat, has some similarities with the grid constructed by Seedhouse (1988) for health promotion. This framework has four layers. The first is concerned with those ethical precepts that allow evaluators to function in the field, whether this is a school, a factory or a community. They are as follows: being sensitive to the needs of participants in the evaluation, even if those needs are not recognized by those participants; assuring their anonymity so that they cannot be identified by other people within or outside the setting since this has the potential to do them harm (again, this might involve evaluators in changing details in the report or omitting information from that report if they feel that it could compromise the interests of participants); and creating a consensual relationship with participants which means that those participants are not compelled to provide them with data (again, this might involve them in deliberately ignoring practice within an institution in which pressures are placed on members of the organization to co-operate with the evaluation).

The second layer is directly epistemological in character. That is, it is concerned with the idea of fidelity and centres round efforts to collect data about the health promotion activity. Evaluators need to collect data which are comprehensive and holistically relate to the setting to avoid partiality. The analysis made of those data must also be faithful to them; that is, the analysis and the theories subsequently developed must be grounded in those data. For example, if evaluators during their fieldwork come across cases or instances which act to disconfirm their theories, then it is important for them to either reject those theories or modify them. Furthermore, this fidelity to the proper relationship between data and analysis applies equally to the relationship between the analysis and any conclusions subsequently drawn. These are epistemological matters; that is, they affect how the evaluator can come to know that reality which they are trying to describe. However, it also refers to the relationship between the methods chosen (i.e. questionnaires, experiments, interviews, observations and documentary analysis) and the deeper ontological relations that persist in social life. This layer is therefore concerned with the choices evaluators make about how they can produce knowledge of the health promotion initiative they are interested in and subsequently about how best they can describe that knowledge in their evaluation reports. In certain circumstances, those precepts located in layer one may be in conflict with those in layer two.

The third layer focuses on the purposes of the health promotion in question. It is important to clarify these purposes to ascertain whether the designers of the programme have created a coherent framework which is likely to improve health in the community. This needs to be understood in two ways: first, whether the notion of a healthy community implied by the initiative is worthwhile and will lead to an increase of individual, group, community and social good; second, whether the idea of health being promoted can be realistically delivered in the way proposed in the project being evaluated. Evaluation cannot simply concern itself with the success or otherwise of the initiative, but must also try to answer ethical, political, philosophical and social questions about the good life with particular reference to health.

The fourth layer is related to this and is concerned with issues of dissemination and change. Questions to be addressed include the following: how and at what stage of the health promotion project should findings be disseminated? How should evaluation reports be constructed and how can writers of them influence the way they are read? Ethical issues are ever present in the inscription process since texts may be constructed in a number of ways. They may be continuous or broken; confessional or

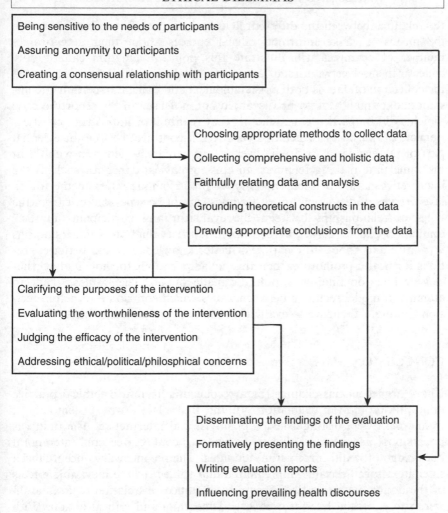

Figure 9.1 Framework for evaluating health promotion.

neutral (Van Maanan, 1988; Usher, 1993); transparent or opaque (Scott, 1996b); 'readerly' or 'writerly' (Barthes, 1975); monologic or dialogic (Hammersley and Atkinson, 1994). All these different textual devices structure the way they can be read and refer to different ways by which evaluators can come to understandings of human activities or, in the case we are referring to here, health promotion activities. These different ways of dissemination and the need to present conclusions as formative have important ethical consequences. The framework is displayed in Figure 9.1.

It is not intended that evaluators of health promotion projects should make ethical decisions by referring to only one layer of the framework. It is the relations between the different layers which provide the evaluator with the means to make informed ethical choices about their activities. A number of examples will illustrate this point. Evaluators cannot only concern themselves with issues of fidelity because, as I have argued above, the collection of data is both epistemological and ethical. In certain circumstances data may have to be discarded and not used in the report because they may harm participants, whether they realize it or not. Again, clarification of the purposes of health education is considered to be an essential part of the evaluator's brief. However, this cannot be achieved without at the same time making reference to epistemological concerns, such as the interpretive nature of social activity. A final example refers to the fourth layer. Issues of dissemination of findings cannot be separated out from the types of relationships between the evaluator and participants in their evaluation that have been agreed upon. If the evaluation is understood as formative and about the creation of better knowledge of and better conditions for health promotion, then this has implications for how and at what stage evaluation findings should be made public. The framework is an attempt to model relations between issues which contribute to better decision making with regard to evaluating health promotion activities.

CONCLUSION

I have argued in this chapter for a reconceptualization of ethical practice in health promotion evaluation. In the first place, two epistemological frameworks were distinguished – positivist and interpretive. The first was understood as offering objective, neutral, context-free and atemporal knowledge of health promotion activities. The second was conceptualized as context specific, value impregnated and subject to the inevitable effects of the double hermeneutic. Three ethical stances in relation to evaluation were subsequently described: covert, democratic and critical action. With regards to the first of these, it was suggested that concealing from participants in evaluation projects knowledge of the purposes of the project would have three consequences: it would diminish or 'dwarf' (Seedhouse, 1988) participants in the evaluation; it would make it more difficult to ascribe generalizability to the findings of the particular case being investigated; and it would restrict the capacity of the evaluators to engage in processes of knowledge construction with participants in the project.

Democratic evaluation, it was suggested, seeks to describe health promotion activities by referencing participants' understandings of their roles and responsibilities within the setting. It was argued that this approach is flawed for three reasons: first, purely phenomenological perspectives ignore the limitations of accounts given by social actors, in that human beings do not and cannot have full knowledge of the perspectives that underlie their everyday actions; second, democratic approaches ignore the possibility that ethical absolutes may be in conflict when applied to health promotion settings; and third, they ignore the nature of evaluation settings, constructed as these are in terms of vested interests, inadequate exchanges of information and differential amounts of power between stakeholders.

Critical action approaches, it was argued, seek to borrow from democratic evaluation many of their central tenets, but to extend them and create a more flexible framework for evaluations. Acknowledging that there is an active element involved in evaluation, critical action theory seeks to tie more closely together epistemological and ethical frameworks, recreate the relationship between evaluators and health promoters so that their roles are intertwined and operate from perspectives which are essentially ethical in orientation. To achieve this, an ethical framework has been developed which is an attempt to both acknowledge the complexity of the evaluation settings and at the same time allow effective decision making by evaluators working in the field.

NOTES

1. Norris (1990) argues that for all practical purposes, evaluation and research are not distinct activities. My argument is based on this same presupposition.
2. Empiricism involves the belief that the only certain knowledge resides in the constant conjunction of observable events or phenomena.
3. Technical rationality or instrumental rational is understood by critical theorists (Marcuse, 1964; Adorno, 1967; Horkheimer, 1972) as the dominant feature of the modern world. They describe it as constraining and distorting and propose solutions which are emancipatory. Gibson (1986:7) describes it in the following way: 'Instrumental rationality represents the preoccupation with means in preference to ends. It is concerned with method and efficiency rather than with purposes. Instrumental rationality limits itself to "How to do it?" questions rather than "Why do it?" or "Where are we going?" questions. It is the divorce of fact from value, and the preference in that divorce, for fact. It is the obsession with calculation and measurement: the drive to classify, to label, to assess and number, all that is human. As such, it is the desire to control and to dominate, to exercise surveillance and power over others and nature'.
4. To use the word 'phenomenology' is not to refer to a single unified body of thought, though its origins can be traced back to Edmund Husserl.
5. Naive realism or representational realism posits an uncomplicated relationship between reality and the way we describe it.

REFERENCES

Adorno, T. (1967) *Prisms: Cultural Criticism and Society*, London: Neville Spearman.

Barthes, R. (1975) *S/Z*, London: Jonathan Cape.

Bkaskar, R. (1979) *The Possibility of Naturalism*, Brighton: Harvester Press.

Bhaskar, R. (1989) *Reclaiming Reality*, London: Verso.

Bracht, G.H. and Glass, G.V. (1968) The external validity of experiments. *American Educational Research Journal*, **4**(5), 437–474.

Burgess, R.G. (1984) *In the Field: An Introduction to Field Relations*, London: Allen and Unwin.

Campbell, D.T. and Stanley, J.C. (1963) Experimental and quasi-experimental designs for research on teaching. In N. Gage (ed.) *Handbook of Research on Teaching*, Chicago: Rand McNally.

Carr, W. and Kemmis, S. (1986) *Becoming Critical: Education, Knowledge and Action Research*, Lewes: Falmer Press.

Carr, W. (1995) *For Education: Towards Critical Educational Inquiry*, Buckingham: Open University.

Denzin, N. (1989) *Interpretive Interactionism, Vol 16, Applied Social Research Methods*, London: Sage.

Gadamer, H.-G. (1975) *Truth and Method*, London: Sheed and Ward.

Gibson, R. (1986) *Critical Theory and Education*, London: Hodder and Stoughton.

Giddens, A. (1984) *The Constitution of Society*, Cambridge: Polity Press.

Guba, E. and Lincoln, Y. (1985) *Naturalistic Inquiry*, London: Sage.

Guba, E. and Lincoln, Y. (1989) *Fourth Generation Evaluation*, London: Sage.

Habermas, J. (1978) *Knowledge and Human Interests*, 2nd edn, London: Heinemann.

Hammersley, M. (1992) *What's Wrong with Ethnography*? London: Routledge.

Hammersley, M. and Atkinson, P. (1994) Ethnography and participant observation. In N. Denzin and Y. Lincoln (eds) *Handbook of Qualitative Research*, London: Sage.

Horkheimer, M. (1972) *Critical Theory: Selected Essays*, New York: Herder and Herder.

Kant, I. (1974–1977) *Works*, Bonn: Suhkamp Taschenbucher.

Marcuse, H. (1964) *One Dimensional Man: Studies in the Ideology of Advanced Industrial Societies*, London: Routledge and Kegan Paul.

Mill, J.S. (1910) *Utilitarianism, Liberty and Representative Government*, London: Dent.

Norris, N. (1990) *Understanding Educational Evaluation*, London: Kogan Page.

Reinharz, S. (1992) *Feminist Methods in Social Research*, New York: Oxford University Press.

Scott, D. (1996a) Methods and data in educational settings. In D. Scott and R. Usher (eds) *Understanding Educational Research*, London: Routledge.

Scott, D. (1996b) Ethnography and education. In D. Scott and R. Usher (eds) *Understanding Educational Research*, London: Routledge.

Seedhouse, D. (1986) *Health: The Foundations of Achievement*, Chichester: Wiley.

Seedhouse, D. (1988) *Ethics: The Heart of Health Care*, Chichester: John Wiley.

Simons, H. (1984) Negotiating conditions for independent evaluations. In C. Adelman (ed.) *The Politics and Ethics of Evaluation*, London: Croom Helm.

Simons, H. (1987) *Getting to Know Schools in a Democracy: The Politics and Process of Evaluation*, London: Falmer Press.

Tones, K. and Tilford, S. (1994) *Health Education: Effectiveness and Efficiency*, 2nd edition, London: Chapman and Hall.

Usher, R. (1993) *Reflexivity*. Occasional Papers in Education as Interdisciplinary Studies, No. 3, Southampton: University of Southampton, School of Education.

Van Maanan, J. (1988) *Tales of the Field: On Writing Ethnography*, Chicago: University of Chicago Press.

<table>
<tr><td>**10**</td><td># Afterword: theory into practice</td></tr>
</table>

10	# Afterword: theory into practice

David Scott and Ros Weston

The various authors in this book have approached the problem of evaluating health promotion in a number of different ways. Weston, for example, uses a postmodern framework, in which the emphasis is on exposing the myth that there is only one type of truth and therefore one type of correct method. Evaluation texts are treated as manifestations of particular power arrangements in society and history and therefore constitutive of the interests of particular groups of people. The implication is that no one particular text is more authoritative than another; indeed, that authorship conveys a spurious universal authority which merely serves to conceal the power plays in which it is positioned. This would seem to suggest the need for epistemological and ontological 'surfacing' by all evaluators. This is justified in two ways. First, it enables the reader/user/stakeholder to understand the type of truth-claims being made and therefore to be in a position to make a judgement about what subsequent actions they should take. Second, it enables the reader to plan subsequent evaluation strategies so that they can fully understand the reflexive nature of what they are doing. This is in contrast to those who operate from a perspective which denotes the universalizing of truth and the ascription of the theory–practice relationship as essentially unproblematic. This relationship, then, is the theme of this afterword.

Practitioners, and this refers to those engaged in health promotion evaluations and others, conceptualize the theory–practice dynamic in a number of distinctive ways.

1. There is a correct method for collecting data about health promotion interventions. This method leads to the creation of objective, value-free

and authoritative knowledge about how health promoters should behave. Practitioners therefore need to 'bracket out' their own values, experiences and preconceptions as being partial, incomplete and subjective and follow the precepts of researchers whose sole purpose is to develop knowledge which is not dependent on local contextual factors.

2. If there is no correct method, but only a set of methods which produce truths of various kinds and are read in different ways depending on the position of the reader, then the practitioner/evaluator has to make a series of decisions about which text is appropriate and which is not. Theory and practice are here being uncoupled. Whether the practitioner works to the prescriptive framework of the theorist will depend on a number of factors, such as whether the values of the theorist and the practitioner are in accord, whether they share the same epistemological framework and, fundamentally, whether solutions are being provided by the theorist to practical problems encountered during the evaluation.

3. A third position is an extension of the logic expressed in 2. Walsh (1993:43) argues that 'this interpretation' of the theory–practice relationship 'turns on the perception that deliberated, thoughtful, practice is not just the target, but is the major source (perhaps the specifying source) of educational theory'. Furthermore, he suggests that 'there is now a growing confidence within these new fields that their kind of theorizing, relating closely and dialectically with practice, is actually the core of educational studies and not just the endpoint of a system for adopting and delivering outside theories'. Note here the rejection of a role in practice for the theorist, operating as they do from the perspective of an outsider. (I should add that Walsh himself is not endorsing such a position, merely describing it.) Various forms of action research (cf. Elliott, 1991) subscribe to this viewpoint.

4. Finally there is a fourth position, which is that the theorist and the practitioner are actually engaged in different activities. This more closely fits with Walsh's view when he argues that the nature of theorizing practice demands the identification of four different discourses, each of which has implicit within it a distinctive way of understanding a practical field such as education and each of which is a legitimate activity. Walsh (1993:44) suggests that there are four mutually supporting kinds of discourse, which he designates as 'deliberation in the strict sense of weighing alternatives and prescribing action in some concrete here and now ... evaluation, also concrete, and at once closely related to deliberation and semi-independent of it ... science, which has a much less direct relationship to practice ... and utopianism, being the form of discourse in which ideal visions and abstract principles are formulated and argued over'. The consequence of this is that the

theorist and the practitioner or, in Walsh's terms, the scientist and the deliberator are operating through different sets of principles and different criteria as to what constitutes knowledge.

Having set out the four positions with little comment, let us now try to make sense of the important relationship under discussion. The first point to make is that 'scientific' theory is designated as theory because relations are being expressed at a general level; that is, they apply to a variety of situations both presently and in the future. They therefore have the power of prediction, not, it should be noted, because the expression of that theory influences what will happen but because the knowledge itself is propositional, generalizable, non-particularistic and operates outside the realm of actual practice. This means that evaluation of health promotion practice is conceived of as the following of rules which have been systematically researched and formalized as theory. Scott, in Chapter 9, refers to the technical-rationality model of the theory–practice relationship in which practice is understood as the practical application of a body of theoretical knowledge. Worthwhile knowledge is seen as being located in the field of generalized propositions, practice is not conceived of as knowledge at all but as the application of theory in practical situations.

This view makes a number of assumptions about the world: first and foremost, that theoretical knowledge can give us insights into reality; that is, it can provide adequate, accurate and meaningful descriptions of how the world works. Second, that practice itself or practical knowledge is not in itself sufficiently organized to qualify as knowledge, i.e. the criteria we apply to something for it to qualify as knowledge (consistency, coherence, validity, reliability and generalizability) cannot apply in practice. Schon (1983) argues that this conception of the theory–practice dynamic cannot itself provide an adequate description of the relationship. Furthermore, because practical knowledge is always considered to be inferior to theoretical knowledge, the privileging of the latter over the former has to be understood as a consequence of history and not as an *a priori* theoretical truth. Schon wants to reconceptualize this power differential and position practical knowledge as knowledge in its own right. This can therefore be contrasted with the technical-rationality model which understands practice as:

> ...the solving of technical problems through rational decision-making procedures based on predictive knowledge. It is the means to achieve ends where the assumption is that ends to which practice is directed can always be predefined and are always knowable. The condition of practice is the learning of a body of theoretical knowledge, and practice therefore becomes the application of this body of knowledge in repeated and predictable ways to achieve predefined ends (Usher *et al.*, 1996: 26).

However, in order for us to follow Schon's reconceptualization of the theory–practice relationship in ways which take it beyond the technical-rationality model, it is important to understand practical knowledge as not being merely the obverse and frequently inferior view of theoretical knowledge. That is, practical knowledge is unsystematic, particularistic, ungeneralizable and located in the here and now.

This is perhaps an appropriate time to return to the continuum developed at the beginning of this afterword in which four positions were distinguished. The third of these understands practice as deliberative action concerned with the making of appropriate decisions about practical problems *in situ*. This does not mean that there is no theoretical activity implicit in the making of these decisions. However, what it does imply is that theoretical activity cannot just apply to technical decisions about how to implement theory developed by outsiders. It is not just that practitioners need to deliberate about the most efficient means to achieve certain predefined ends, it is those ends themselves which are subject to the deliberative process. As Schon suggests, practice situations are not only particularistic, 'they are also characterized by a complexity and uncertainty which resist routinization' (Usher *et al.*, 1996: 127). They need to undergo continual processes of renewal. In short, such knowledge is performative rather than propositional, which means that there is always an action component to practice.

Adopting this standpoint leaves us with a number of problems. By relegating external theory, or science as Walsh calls it, to a different realm, the relationship between theory and practice becomes more opaque. Second, this new and more distant relationship between theory and practice has certain consequences. The difficulty is to conceptualize it without resorting to timeless truths about evaluation. Operating in a non-technicist way demands that practitioners do not behave as objective theorists say they should. But this reconceptualizing of the relationship between theory and practice is itself theoretical and, moreover, theoretical in a normative sense. This can only be resolved by accepting the need for theoretical knowledge, which means that it has to refer to something. This is indeed Usher *et al.*'s solution as they accept that there is a place for theory in practical discourse, which of course closely ties together theory and practice. For them, informal theory central to practice 'is situated theory both entering into and emerging from practice' (Usher *et al.*, 1996: 35).

What, then, is the role of the evaluator of health promotion projects? Our notional practitioner, the health promoter, has certain definite ends in mind and carries them with her to the evaluation. The evaluator is concerned with the assessment of the effectiveness or otherwise of particular projects or interventions. However, what has been stressed repeatedly throughout this book is that the evaluator's toolkit for the making of such judgements is not and cannot be merely a neutral set of criteria. Those criteria are underpinned by a view of both how the world works and how we can know it. In other words, evaluators, whether they acknowledge it or not, are always positioned within ontological and epistemological frameworks.

The problems this creates for achieving agreement about effectiveness (cf. Fraser, 1996) have led some (Tones, 1996, and in this book) to argue for a notion of judicial review. Evidence, for him, would be judged sufficient if it was enough to convince a notional jury that it was compelling and, indeed, compelling enough to allow them to commit themselves to action. In other words, there are no absolute standards of proof which can be applied. This allows a further way for informal theory to enter into and inform practice. If the practitioner acting as a notional member of a jury judges the knowledge procured from evaluation sufficiently compelling in a practical sense, then use can be made of it. This both informs and enriches theory and practice, in particular as it relates to the development of a healthier society.

REFERENCES

Elliott, J. (1991) *Action Research for Educational Change*, Milton Keynes: Open University Press.

Fraser, E. (1996) Guest editorial: how effective are effectiveness reviews? *Health Education Journal*, **55**, 359–362.

Schon, D. (1983) *The Reflective Practitioner: How Professionals Think in Action*, Aldershot: Avebury.

Tones, K. (1996) Conflict and compromise in health promotion research: a quest for illumination. Paper given at the Conference on the Status of Nordic Health Promotion Research, Bergen, August.

Usher, R., Bryant, I. and Johnston, R. (1996) *Adult Education and the Post-Modern Challenge: Learning beyond the Limits*, London: Routledge.

Walsh, P. (1993) *Education and Meaning: Philosophy in Practice*, London: Cassell.

Author Index

Subject Index